Advance praise for *Applications of the Unified Protocols for Transdiagnostic Treatment of Emotional Disorders in Children and Adolescents*

"The unified protocol features a single set of cognitive behavioral principles applicable to the full range of disorders of emotion. Nowhere is this more starkly illustrated than in this important book from Jill Ehrenreich-May and Sarah M. Kennedy. From tic/Tourette disorder to pediatric disruptive mood dysregulation disorder clinicians will learn the art of applying this one set of common principles to the full range of emotional disorders in children and adolescents. Every clinician working with this population should have this book handy."

—**David H. Barlow**, PhD, ABPP, Professor of Psychology and
Psychiatry Emeritus, Founder, Center for Anxiety and
Related Disorders (CARD), Boston University

"This comprehensive volume brings the delivery of the Unified Protocols for Children and Adolescents to life with rich case examples and extensive practical knowledge. In particular, the focused nature of the chapters and straightforward tip sheets will make this work an invaluable guide for busy clinicians (and trainees) interested in implementing a single, streamlined intervention to the vast majority of mental health difficulties faced by youth."

—**Shannon Sauer-Zavala**, PhD, Department of Psychology,
University of Kentucky

ABCT Clinical Practice Series

Series Editor

Susan W. White, Ph.D., ABPP, Professor and Doddridge Saxon Chair in Clinical Psychology, University of Alabama

Associate Editors

Lara J. Farrell, Ph.D., Associate Professor, School of Applied Psychology, Griffith University & Menzies Health Institute of Queensland, Australia

Matthew A. Jarrett, Ph.D., Associate Professor, Department of Psychology, University of Alabama

Jordana Muroff, Ph.D., LICSW, Associate Professor, Clinical Practice, Boston University School of Social Work

Marisol Perez, Ph.D., Associate Professor & Associate Chair, Department of Psychology, Arizona State University

Titles in the Series

Applications of the Unified Protocol for Transdiagnostic Treatment of Emotional Disorders
Edited by David H. Barlow and Todd Farchione

Helping Families of Youth with School Attendance Problems
Christopher A. Kearney

Addressing Parental Accommodation When Treating Anxiety in Children
Eli R. Lebowitz

Exposure Therapy for Eating Disorders
Carolyn Black Becker, Nicholas R. Farrell, and Glenn Waller

Exposure Therapy for Child and Adolescent Anxiety and OCD
Stephen P. H. Whiteside, Thomas H. Ollendick, and Bridget K. Biggs

Managing Microaggressions
Monnica T. Williams

A Clinician's Guide to Disclosures of Sexual Assault
Amie R. Newins and Laura C. Wilson

Applications of the Unified Protocols for Transdiagnostic Treatment of Emotional Disorders in Children and Adolescents

EDITED BY

JILL EHRENREICH-MAY

AND

SARAH M. KENNEDY

OXFORD
UNIVERSITY PRESS

OXFORD
UNIVERSITY PRESS

Oxford University Press is a department of the University of Oxford. It furthers
the University's objective of excellence in research, scholarship, and education
by publishing worldwide. Oxford is a registered trade mark of Oxford University
Press in the UK and certain other countries.

Published in the United States of America by Oxford University Press
198 Madison Avenue, New York, NY 10016, United States of America.

© Oxford University Press 2021

Library of Congress Cataloging-in-Publication Data
Names: Ehrenreich-May, Jill, editor. | M. Kennedy, Sarah, editor.
Title: Applications of the unified protocols for transdiagnostic treatment
of emotional disorders in children and adolescents / Jill Ehrenreich-May
and Sarah M. Kennedy.
Description: New York, NY : Oxford University Press, [2021] |
Series: ABCT clinical practice series | Includes bibliographical references and index.
Identifiers: LCCN 2021015053 (print) | LCCN 2021015054 (ebook) |
ISBN 9780197527931 (paperback) | ISBN 9780197527894 (epub) |
ISBN 9780197527900
Subjects: LCSH: Child psychotherapy. | Adolescent psychotherapy.
Classification: LCC RJ504 .A67 2021 (print) | LCC RJ504 (ebook) |
DDC 618.92/8914—dc23
LC record available at https://lccn.loc.gov/2021015053
LC ebook record available at https://lccn.loc.gov/2021015054

DOI: 10.1093/med-psych/9780197527931.001.0001

9 8 7 6 5 4 3 2 1

Printed by Marquis, Canada

CONTENTS

Part 3 Adapting the UP-C and UP-A to Different Treatment Settings

Mental health clinicians desperately want to help their clients, and recognize the importance of implementing evidence-based treatments toward achieving this goal. In the past several years, the field of mental health care has seen tremendous advances in our understanding of pathology and its underlying mechanisms, as well as proliferation and refinement of scientifically informed treatment approaches. Coinciding with these advances is a heightened focus on accountability in clinical practice. Clinicians are expected to apply evidence-based approaches, and to do so effectively, efficiently, and in a client-centered, individualized way. This is no small order. For a multitude of reasons, including but not limited to client diversity, complex psychopathology (e.g., comorbidity), and barriers to care that are not under the clinician's control (e.g., adverse life circumstances that limit the client's ability to participate), delivery of evidence-based approaches can be challenging.

This series, which represents a collaborative effort between the Association for Behavioral and Cognitive Therapies (ABCT) and the Oxford University Press, is intended to serve as an easy-to-use, highly practical collection of resources for clinicians and trainees. The *ABCT Clinical Practice Series* is designed to help clinicians effectively master and implement evidence-based treatment approaches. In practical terms, the series represents the "brass tacks" of implementation, including basic how-to guidance and advice on troubleshooting common issues in clinical practice and application. As such, the series is best viewed as a complement to other series on evidence-based protocols such as the *Treatments That Work*™ series and the *Programs That Work*™ series. These represent seminal bridges between research and practice and have been instrumental in the dissemination of empirically supported intervention protocols and programs. The *ABCT Clinical Practice Series*, rather than focusing on specific diagnoses and their treatment, targets the practical application of therapeutic and assessment approaches. In other words, the emphasis is on the *how-to* aspects of mental health delivery.

It is my hope that clinicians and trainees find these books useful in refining their clinical skills, as enhanced comfort as well as competence in delivery of evidence-based approaches should ultimately lead to improved client outcomes. Given the emphasis on application in this series, there is relatively less emphasis on review of the underlying research base. Readers who wish to delve more deeply into the theoretical or empirical basis supporting specific approaches are encouraged to go to the original source publications cited in each chapter. When relevant, suggestions for further reading are provided.

One of the most firmly established tenets of child clinical psychology is that comorbidity is the rule, not the exception. This fact can make selection of a disorder-focused treatment approach challenging. Transdiagnostic treatments seek to address underlying processes that give rise to a range of manifest problems across domains—behavior, socialization, and emotion. The Unified Protocols for Transdiagnostic Treatment of Emotional Disorders in Children and Adolescents (UP-C and UP-A) address core dysfunction areas, such as neuroticism, distress intolerance, and behavioral avoidance, to improve functioning and reduce symptoms in clients. The UP-A and UP-C have a rich empirical base that supports their use with a range of disorders and presenting problems.

This book, *Applications of the Unified Protocols for Transdiagnostic Treatment of Emotional Disorders in Children and Adolescents*, supplements the published UP-C and UP-A manuals (Ehrenreich-May et al., 2018) by providing practical guidance for clinicians treating the full range of psychopathology in youth. This volume unpacks key distinctions of the different techniques employed in the UP-C/A and explains adaptations for different problem areas. Whether the reader is experienced in using the UP-C/A or is a novice to this approach, this book can be a useful hands-on resource.

Dr. Jill Ehrenreich-May and Dr. Sarah M. Kennedy are experts in clinical child psychology and certified trainers for the UP-C/A. In this volume, along with their co-authors, they draw on their years of expertise gleaned from research and clinical experience working with children and adolescents to provide extremely useful guidance on application of the UP-C/A.

Susan W. White, PhD, ABPP
Series Editor

REFERENCE

Ehrenreich-May, J., Kennedy, S. M., Sherman, J. A., Bilek, E. L., Buzzella, B. A., Bennett, S. M., & Barlow, D. H. (2018). *Unified protocols for transdiagnostic treatment of emotional disorders in children and adolescents: Therapist guide.* Oxford University Press.

CONTRIBUTORS

Jafar Bakhshaie, MD, PhD
Department of Psychiatry
Massachusetts General Hospital/
 Harvard Medical School

Dylan Braun, MS
College of Psychology
Nova Southeastern University

**Renee L. Brown, BPsySci(Hons),
MPsych(Clin)**
School of Psychology
University of Queensland

**Vanessa E. Cobham, PhD
(Clin Psych)**
School of Psychology
University of Queensland

Kristina Duncombe Lowe, PhD
Children's MN Center for the
 Treatment of Eating Disorders

Sarah Eckhardt, PhD
Children's MN Center for the
 Treatment of Eating Disorders

Jill Ehrenreich-May, PhD
Department of Psychology
University of Miami

Corinne A. Elmore, PhD
Department of Health Psychology
Walter Reed National Military
 Medical Center

Rebecca E. Ford-Paz, PhD
Pritzker Department of Psychiatry and
 Behavioral Health
Ann & Robert H. Lurie Children's
 Hospital of Chicago, Northwestern
 University Feinberg School of
 Medicine

Hiroko Fujisato, PhD
Department of Preventive Intervention
 for Psychiatric Disorders, National
 Institute of Mental Health
National Center of Neurology and
 Psychiatry

Rinatte Gruen, BA
Department of Psychology
University of Miami

Elizabeth R. Halliday, BS
Department of Psychology
University of Miami

Jessica Lyn Hawks, PhD
Department of Psychiatry; Pediatric
 Mental Health Institute
University of Colorado; Children's
 Hospital Colorado

**Jacob Benjamin Westrick
Holzman, PhD**
Department of Psychiatry
University of Colorado Anschutz
 School of Medicine

Judy H. Hong, PhD
Louis A. Faillace, MD, Department of
    Psychiatry and Behavioral Sciences
University of Texas Health
    Science Center

Noriko Kato, PhD
Department of Neuropsychiatry
Keio University School of Medicine

Sarah M. Kennedy, PhD
Department of Psychiatry
University of Colorado Anschutz
    School of Medicine

Ryan R. Landoll, PhD, MHPE, ABPP
Office for Student Affairs
Uniformed Services University of the
    Health Sciences

Vanesa A. Mora Ringle, PhD
The Penn Collaborative for CBT and
    Implementation Science
University of Pennsylvania

Dominique Phillips, BS
Department of Psychology
University of Miami

Estefany Sáez-Clarke, MS
Department of Psychology
University of Miami

Alison Salloum, PhD, LCSW
Department of School of Social Work
University of South Florida

Ashley M. Shaw, PhD
Center for Children and Families
Florida International University

Eric A. Storch, PhD
Department of Psychiatry and
    Behavioral Sciences
Baylor College of Medicine

**Kade B. Thornton, ENS (Military
Rank), BS**
Department of Medical and Clinical
    Psychology
Uniformed Services University of the
    Health Sciences

Niza Tonarely, PhD
Department of Psychology
University of Miami

Thanh T. Truong, MD
Department of Psychiatry and
    Behavioral Sciences
Baylor College of Medicine

Jason Washburn, PhD
Department of Psychiatry and
    Behavioral Sciences
Northwestern University

Marc J. Weintraub, PhD
Department of Psychiatry
UCLA Semel Institute

Faith Summersett Williams, PhD
Department of Psychiatry and
    Behavioral Sciences and
    Department of Pediatrics
Northwestern University Feinberg
    School of Medicine

Jamie Zinberg, MA
Semel Institute for Neuroscience and
    Human Behavior
University of California

PART 1

An Evidence-Based Approach to Working with Youths

Introduction to the Unified Protocols for Transdiagnostic Treatment of Emotional Disorders in Children and Adolescents

History, Rationale, Adaptations

SARAH M. KENNEDY AND JILL EHRENREICH-MAY ■

HISTORY OF TRANSDIAGNOSTIC TREATMENTS

The Unified Protocols for Transdiagnostic Treatment of Emotional Disorders in Children and Adolescents (UP-C/UP-A; Ehrenreich-May et al., 2018) are transdiagnostic interventions designed to address multiple diagnoses, diagnostic categories, and/or problem types within a single treatment protocol. It might be said that modern transdiagnostic interventions originated within the early years of the 21st century with theoretical and empirical work by Barlow and colleagues conceptualizing a "unified approach" to understanding and treating emotional disorders (e.g., Barlow et al., 2004) and, subsequently, the initial publication of the Unified Protocols for Transdiagnostic Treatment of Emotional Disorders (Barlow et al., 2011). However, up until the mid-20th century, psychotherapeutic approaches were nothing if not transdiagnostic, in that they addressed underlying psychodynamic and interpersonal processes theorized to lead to the development of broad psychological neuroses. This approach changed during the second half of the 20th century, in accordance with two parallel and mutually informative developments.

First, with each new iteration of the American Psychiatric Association (APA)'s *Diagnostic and Statistical Manual of Mental Disorders* (DSM) from the publication of the original DSM in 1952 to DSM-IV in 1994, the number of diagnoses proliferated, and diagnostic criteria became increasingly fine-grained. During the same historical period, new treatments for these highly specified diagnoses were developed based on new empirical and theoretical evidence (e.g., exposure for phobias), and more rigorous outcomes research on cognitive-behavioral therapy (CBT) and other interventions began to emerge (Barlow et al., 2004). Psychotherapy research was conducted using newly developed treatment manuals addressing symptoms of highly specific diagnoses (e.g., panic disorder, specific phobias) to help ensure scientific rigor and replicability. The turn back toward transdiagnostic models of psychopathology and treatment at the turn of the 21st century was based on growing recognition of the commonalities among psychiatric diagnoses, the shared features of psychotherapeutic interventions for distinct diagnoses, and the beneficial effects of treatments for one diagnosis on other diagnoses, which will be further discussed later in the chapter.

While this story accurately describes the evolution from diagnosis-specific interventions to transdiagnostic interventions for adult psychopathology, the evolution for child and adolescent (hereafter referred to together as "youth") interventions differs somewhat in its steps. Prior to the late 1980s and early 1990s, psychodynamic therapies such as play therapy were the primary modality in youth treatment. Early studies of behavioral and cognitive-behavioral interventions for childhood phobias appeared in the 1980s but were generally small and uncontrolled and targeted very specific fears or clinical presentations (Benjamin et al., 2011). Here the history of interventions for child psychopathology diverges from that of interventions for adult psychopathology, as some of the earliest randomized trials of treatments for youth problems can be conceptualized as, at least to some extent, transdiagnostic. The first randomized clinical trial of CBT for anxiety, for example, was transdiagnostic across a subset of anxiety disorders (e.g., generalized anxiety disorder, separation anxiety disorder, and social anxiety disorder; Kendall, 1994). With regard to externalizing disorders in childhood, Patterson's work on factors contributing to the emergence and maintenance of aggressive and problem behaviors, including coercive interactions between caregivers and children (Patterson, 1982), led to the development of parent management training approaches for addressing disruptive behaviors. While there are certainly numerous treatment manuals for youth with specific disorders, several early interventions that gained empirical support focused on disorder classes or more broad problem areas, rather than narrow slices of psychopathology.

The emergence of transdiagnostic interventions for youth that cut across problem areas or disorder classes occurred somewhat in parallel with the emergence of adult transdiagnostic interventions. Chorpita et al. (2005) proposed a "distillation and matching model," whereby interventions were reconceptualized not on the level of the treatment manual but rather on the level of individual components referred to as "practice elements," therapeutic interventions common across evidence-based treatments. Practice elements could then be "matched," or arranged and selected according to client or contextual factors based on decision trees or algorithms. The distillation and matching approach gave rise to the Modular Approach to Therapy for Children with Anxiety, Depression, or Conduct Problems (MATCH; Chorpita et al., 2013; Weisz et al., 2012), one of the first "modular" transdiagnostic treatments for youth composed of practice elements addressing anxiety, depression, disruptive conduct symptoms, and traumatic stress symptoms in youth. Some, more recent youth transdiagnostic treatments take a "principle-guided approach" based on identification of a limited set of therapeutic change processes, rather than individual treatment components, common across evidence-based treatments for youth. The FIRST protocol (Weisz et al., 2017), for example, contains five therapeutic principles of change (e.g., increasing motivation, repairing thoughts) designed to be flexibly delivered to address youth anxiety, depression, and conduct problems.

The UP-A, developed to some extent in tandem with MATCH, is a downward adaptation of the adult UP that takes what has been referred to as a "core-dysfunction–based" approach to youth transdiagnostic treatment (Marchette & Weisz, 2017), in contrast to the modular approach taken by MATCH. Core-dysfunction–based approaches to youth emotional disorders address multiple forms of psychopathology and comorbidity among diagnoses by targeting underlying dysfunctions apparently shared across psychopathology. For example, both the adult and youth UPs address the core dysfunction of engagement in maladaptive action tendencies, such as behavioral avoidance, by promoting more approach-oriented and adaptive actions through such strategies as acting "opposite" to maladaptive action tendencies and exposure. Other core-dysfunction-based approaches to treating youth include group behavioral activation therapy (Chu et al., 2009), which targets behavioral avoidance common across youth anxiety and depression, and the Coping Cat-based EMOTION prevention program, which targets avoidance and maladaptive cognitions (Martinsen et al., 2016). The UP-C and UP-A may also be contrasted with principle-guided approaches such as FIRST. As noted earlier, FIRST is organized around a set of five therapeutic principles common among evidence-based treatments (EBTs) for youth internalizing and externalizing disorders, presented in an easily digestible, transdiagnostic format. Although the UP-C and UP-A certainly contain therapeutic principles or intervention strategies recognizable from other EBTs, the UP-C and UP-A employ such strategies to address underlying core dysfunctions thought to be modifiable treatment targets. In the following sections, we discuss how core UP-C and UP-A intervention strategies are designed to modify such targets.

The UP-A was first developed as a downward adaptation of the adult UP that presented a similar set of intervention techniques to address core dysfunctions in a developmentally appropriate format, using adolescent-friendly language and examples and incorporating caregivers through an additional "Module P" (Ehrenreich et al., 2009). The development of the UP-C further extended UP principles addressing underlying core dysfunctions of emotional disorders to children ages six to 12 by further enhancing parent involvement, adapting treatment delivery and materials for elementary-age children, and increasing the experiential and interactive emphasis of treatment (Ehrenreich-May & Bilek, 2012). As with all good treatments, these protocols have been revised over the years based on research findings (discussed in Chapter 3 of this volume) and feedback from families and clinicians, resulting in the publication of the *Unified Protocols for Transdiagnostic Treatment of Emotional Disorders in Children and Adolescents: Therapist Guide* in 2017 (Ehrenreich-May et al., 2018). Chapter 2 of this volume provides an overview of the standard delivery format of UP-C and UP-A for the treatment of anxiety and depressive disorders.

RATIONALE FOR TRANSDIAGNOSTIC TREATMENT OF EMOTIONAL DISORDERS

The development of transdiagnostic treatments over the past several decades has been motivated by the oft-cited observation that comorbidity among emotional disorders is the rule rather than the exception. Indeed, up to two-thirds of clinic-referred youth with a primary anxiety diagnosis receive at least one additional diagnosis, with other anxiety disorders being the most common comorbid conditions (Angold et al., 1999). Rates of comorbidity between anxiety and depressive disorders have also been observed to be as high as 75% in some and appear to be particularly elevated in youth with a primary depression diagnosis (Axelson & Birmaher, 2001; Garber & Weersing, 2010; Ollendick et al., 2008). These observations, in addition to findings that youth receiving treatment for an anxiety disorder experience improvements in their depression symptoms, and vice versa (Chu & Harrison, 2007; Suveg et al., 2009; Weisz et al., 2006), suggest that emotional disorders may share risk and maintaining factors, or "core dysfunctions." Addressing these core dysfunctions may be a more parsimonious and effective way of treating emotional disorders, rather than targeting individual symptom clusters.

Despite the potential reduction in training burden, increased cost-effectiveness, and appeal of using a single treatment to target transdiagnostic factors across emotional disorders, we would be remiss not to acknowledge that our current diagnostic system and reimbursement structure incentivizes clinicians to think in terms of diagnosis. Indeed, as mentioned previously, the fifth edition of DSM (DSM-5; APA, 2013) contains more diagnoses than any previous edition, and diagnostic information is still widely employed to guide treatment decisions. Further, clients and families often present for treatment seeking diagnostic information to better understand themselves and/or their child and clarify appropriate treatment decisions. While we would certainly encourage clinicians to think transdiagnostically with case conceptualization and treatment planning by considering how any individual client presents with respect to the core dysfunctions discussed below, we do not believe that diagnosis-based conceptualizations of emotional disorders are inherently in conflict with a transdiagnostic approach. Rather, diagnostic information can be useful in helping clinicians consider which core dysfunctions may be most relevant for a given client; in elucidating how core dysfunctions may manifest differently across clients; and in informing decisions about how to adapt treatment, considering the treatment structure of diagnosis-specific manuals. Readers will notice that many of the chapters in this volume are organized around diagnoses for all of the reasons mentioned above, and others.

That being said, it is our experience that many clinicians in community, school, pediatric, and brief treatment settings may need to arrive at a diagnostic impression for the purpose of billing or documentation, but may not have adequate time or information to draw precise diagnostic conclusions or make complex differential diagnoses. A transdiagnostic approach to treatment may seem quite natural to clinicians in these settings, who may approach treatment from a more problem-focused rather than a diagnosis-focused orientation.

To help clinicians begin conceptualizing cases from a core-dysfunction–based approach, whether in addition to or in place of a diagnostic one, in what follows we briefly discuss some key core dysfunctions underlying emotional disorders. Although a comprehensive discussion of candidate core dysfunctions underlying emotional disorders is beyond the scope of this introduction, we summarize research into several areas most relevant to the UP-C and UP-A.

Neuroticism

Neuroticism, or the trait-like propensity to experience elevated negative affect (NA), is a core underlying feature of emotional disorders supported through genetic findings, behavioral neuroscience, and structural modeling. Clark and Watson's (1991) tripartite model, which has now been extensively evaluated in both youth and adults, proposed that increased NA is a shared process that accounts for symptom overlap and comorbidity among anxiety and depressive disorders, while low positive affect differentiates depressive from anxiety disorders, and increased physiological reactivity differentiates anxiety from depressive disorders. Several studies have supported this three-factor model of emotional disorders in youth (e.g., Chorpita et al., 2000; Laurent et al., 2004). Findings from behavioral neuroscience have also supported the hypothesis that individuals with both anxiety and depressive disorders have a propensity to experience increased levels of negative emotion relative to individuals without an emotional disorder, as well as decreased activity in areas of the frontal lobe associated with inhibition of NA (Wilamowska et al., 2010). Indeed, in our clinical experiences in treating youth with emotional disorders, we have often observed that these youth experience more frequent and intense negative emotions of all sorts (e.g., anxiety, worry, anger, sadness), and many parents describe their children and adolescents as experiencing these difficulties as far back as they can recall.

Distress Intolerance and Aversive Reactions to Emotion

While youth with emotional disorders experience elevated NA compared to youth without emotional disorders, research and our clinical experiences indicate that is often the youth's response to their emotional experience, rather than the emotion itself, that is most impairing. Distress tolerance (DT) is the perceived capacity to handle uncomfortable emotional experiences and persist with goal-directed activities in the face of distress (Zvolensky et al., 2010). Believing that one is unable to handle emotional experiences may increase risk for emotional disorders by increasing the intensity and frequency of the emotion, interfere with ability to focus on social or educational pursuits while experiencing strong emotion, and lead to problematic attempts to dampen or escape the emotion. Indeed, poor DT has been associated with anxiety and depression symptoms in youth (Bardeen et al., 2013; Cummings et al., 2013), and DT has been found to improve with treatment in adults and to be associated with improvements in depression symptoms (McHugh et al., 2013; Williams et al., 2013). In our own research, we have found that youth profiles characterized by poorer DT are associated with higher impairment and slower treatment gains (Kennedy et al., under review). The UP-C and UP-A aim to improve youths' ability to tolerate distress by modifying these distress reactions through the use of mindfulness and nonjudgmental awareness techniques during sensational exposures, "acting opposite" exercises, and exposures designed to elicit a range of emotions.

Information Processing Biases and Cognitive Styles

Youth with emotional disorders have been shown to demonstrate biases in their interpretation of information, as well as cognitive styles that make it difficult for them to reappraise or disengage from unhelpful patterns of thinking. Youth with depression symptoms have been shown to demonstrate a tendency to attend to negative information (e.g., words, faces) and to interpret ambiguous information negatively (Platt et al., 2017). Similarly, evidence indicates that youth with anxiety selectively attend to threat and interpret ambiguous situations as threatening (Bar-Haim et al., 2007; Cannon & Weems, 2010). Perseverative thinking styles common to youth with emotional disorders may in turn create difficulties disengaging from negative or threat-related information once these biases are activated, increasing distress related to these thinking styles. Youth with anxiety and depression have been demonstrated to engage in repetitive negative thinking (RNT) such as rumination and worry, cognitive styles that may increase risk for future symptoms (Hankin, 2008; McLaughlin & Nolen-Hoeksema, 2011), Conversely, youth with emotional disorders may use purportedly adaptive strategies, such as cognitive reappraisal, infrequently and/or ineffectively (Gross & Thompson, 2007). Anxious and depressed youth may also be less likely to engage in helpful cognitive strategies for regulating their emotions, such as reappraising threatening or negative information (e.g., Carthy et al., 2010). Module 5 of the UP-A and Sessions 5 through 7 of the UP-C address these information processing biases and unhelpful cognitive styles by teaching youth to recognize "thinking traps" and to engage in reappraisal strategies to promote more flexible thinking. Additionally, Module 6 of the UP-A and Session 8 of the UP-C, through their focus on present-moment and nonjudgmental awareness, can be used to help youth develop awareness of patterns of RNT and learn to more flexibly focus their attention on aspects of the present moment. Some may argue that there is an uneasy tension between teaching aspects of both cognitive reappraisal and mindfulness in the same intervention. However, understanding that reappraisal is a skill best applied in the antecedent condition, whereas present-moment and nonjudgmental awareness strategies could be applied during any phase of an emotional response, may be a useful framework for understanding the relative utility of each strategy from a temporal standpoint.

Cognitive and Behavioral Avoidance

Youth with emotional disorders often engage in avoidant strategies to regulate their emotions, including cognitive avoidance (e.g., suppressing or distracting from uncomfortable aspects of an emotional experience) or behavioral avoidance (e.g., withdrawing from or avoiding situations or individuals that elicit emotional experiences). These avoidant strategies often become reinforced over time, in that they often provide some immediate short-term relief from the uncomfortable emotion. However, they may maintain or even increase NA in the longer term, may prevent youth from correcting cognitive biases about avoided stimuli or learn that they can tolerate emotional distress, and may limit access to positively reinforcing activities or social opportunities (Campbell-Sills & Barlow, 2007). In this way, cognitive and behavioral avoidance may increase symptoms of anxiety and depression over time. The UP-C and UP-A promote the use of more approach-oriented actions in response to emotional experiences, such as "acting opposite" and exposure, and reinforce mindful and nonjudgmental awareness of emotional experiences as an antidote to cognitive avoidance.

Parenting

The UP-C and UP-A also address several parenting behaviors that have been broadly linked with the development of emotional disorders in youth. Parenting styles characterized by low levels of warmth and high levels of rejection and/or criticism have been associated with the development of both anxiety and depressive disorders (Drake & Ginsburg, 2012). Similarly, overprotective parenting styles and high levels of parent accommodation, or anticipation and prevention of situations that elicit strong emotions, have been linked with anxiety and obsessive-compulsive disorders in youth (Drake & Ginsburg, 2012; Thompson-Hollands et al., 2014). Parents of youth with emotional disorders, who themselves are more likely than parents of healthy youth to have emotional disorders or elevated symptoms themselves, may also model unhelpful responses to strong emotions, such as negative reactions to their own emotional experiences and avoidant regulation strategies. Indeed, several studies have found associations between parent engagement in avoidant strategies such as suppression and increased youth emotional lability and poor emotion regulation (Bariola et al., 2012; Rogers et al., 2016). In both the UP-C and UP-A, parents are introduced to these "emotional behaviors" and learn to replace them with "opposite" or more helpful parenting behaviors, in addition to receiving support in consistently reinforcing their youth's use of skills.

WHY AND WHEN TO ADAPT THE UP-C AND UP-A FOR OTHER POPULATIONS

In general, our clinical, consulting, and research experiences have informed us that using the UP-C and UP-A in their standard, as-written formats generally works well for treating almost all anxiety and depressive disorders (e.g., social anxiety disorder, generalized anxiety disorder, panic disorder, depressive disorders). In the UP-C and UP-A therapist guides, informative "Therapist Notes" draw the therapist's attention to how certain materials may be frontloaded, slightly adapted, or enhanced in order to increase their relevance and impact for youth with varying anxiety and mood presentations. For example, in Module 3 we provide suggestions for how to incorporate exposures earlier in treatment for youth with significant anxiety-related avoidance and readiness to engage in earlier exposure practice, as well as how to engage depressed youth in ongoing activation experiments throughout treatment. In Module 4, we describe how interoceptive or sensational exposures can be enhanced and assigned on an ongoing basis for youth with panic disorder or panic-like symptoms. Such adaptations are relatively minor and, in general, can be easily and intuitively incorporated into standard delivery of UP-C and UP-A.

While the UP-C and UP-A were initially and are perhaps most often used to treat anxiety and depressive disorders, expanding conceptualizations of an "emotional disorder" have increased interest in using these interventions to treat youth with a wider symptom or diagnostic profile. In our experience the core intervention components contained in the UP-C and UP-A are flexible enough to be extended to other symptom or diagnostic profiles, and emerging pilot work, secondary data analyses, and initial results from larger trials support this. However, these applications often require adapting existing UP-C and/or UP-A materials to fit these different symptom presentations and/or delivery settings, and discussion of such adaptations is beyond the scope of the UP-C and UP-A therapist guides and workbooks. Accordingly, we have put this volume together to provide guidance to the clinician wishing to capitalize on the flexibility of the UP-C and UP-A by applying these interventions to youth with symptoms beyond anxiety and depression, and in delivery settings that may not be conducive to the standard weekly therapy approach. This volume also complements Barlow and Farchione's (2017)

Applications of the Unified Protocol for Transdiagnostic Treatment of Emotional Disorders, a clinician resource that illustrates the application of the adult UP to varying clinical presentations, delivery formats, and cultures. It should be mentioned that the chapters in this volume reflect completed and ongoing research on extending the UP-C and UP-A for use with different populations; the UP-C and the UP-A may also be appropriate for other clinical populations or in other contexts, but work in these areas is forthcoming.

What might guide clinical decision-making about for whom the UP-C and UP-A are appropriate? To return to the conceptualization developed previously in this chapter, an emotional disorder is a disorder characterized by (1) frequent, intense experience of negative emotions; (2) distress in response to that emotional experience and perceived inability to tolerate or manage that distress; and (3) use of emotion regulation strategies to manage negative emotions that are either broadly ineffective or provide short-term relief but long-term impairment and exacerbation of the emotional experience. There is growing appreciation of the idea that these criteria apply to non-anxiety and non-mood disorders, including eating disorders, borderline personality disorder or features, obsessive-compulsive disorder, and disorders of childhood characterized primarily by irritability and/or anger, such as disruptive mood dysregulation disorder and intermittent explosive disorder. At the same time, some adaptations may need to be made to the content, format, materials, or order of delivery of therapeutic techniques to optimally address these emotional disorder presentations using the UP-C and UP-A. Chapters 4 through 9 of this volume each focus on adapting the UP-C and/or UP-A for specific diagnoses or symptom presentations that align with this conceptualization of emotional disorders, but that also require some adjustment in the delivery of treatment.

Chapters 10 through 12 turn toward adapting the UP-C and the UP-A to enhance fit with different delivery settings, formats, or cultural contexts. The UP-A was originally designed to be delivered individually to adolescents in standard, 45- or 60-minute weekly sessions, while the UP-C was developed for delivery in a group format with weekly sessions. Both interventions were also initially examined in university-based clinic settings. The UP-C can be easily adapted for individual therapy sessions, as described in Chapter 2. However, many youth do not encounter treatment in this traditional format and may complete a shorter duration of treatment, may access services via telehealth due to location convenience, or may be served in community mental health settings where clinicians are faced with larger caseloads, less time for preparation or training, and more heterogenous client populations. Chapter 10 focuses on adapting the UP-C and UP-A for stepped care delivery via telehealth, while Chapter 11 illustrates how the UP-A may be applied in community mental health settings, based on experiences from two randomized effectiveness trials in the United States and Australia. Finally, given growing interest in the Unified Protocols across the globe and the need for cultural and linguistic adaptations of these interventions, Chapter 12 focuses on efforts to adapt the UP-C for delivery with youth in Japan to illustrate one example of a culturally sensitive adaptation.

FUTURE DIRECTIONS

When training new clinicians to use the UP-C and UP-A, Dr. Ehrenreich-May has often told the story that while the youth version of the UP developed from the primary influence of Dr. Barlow's concurrent work with adults and the theoretical models described earlier in the chapter, it also developed in part out of her own clinical practice with youth and families. In an effort to provide the most flexible and useful version of effective child therapy with these clients, she would often look for the best example of an existent CBT technique or a mindfulness technique, make her own worksheet for it, and flexibly adapt it to fit child or caregiver needs in the moment. In reality, this is what the UP-C and UP-A are at heart—simply a "greatest hits" collection of child-focused behavior therapy strategies brought together for pragmatic purposes, but not truly meant to be used without consideration of the context of the client in front of you. We hope that you find this book inspires good, flexible application of the principles, materials, and techniques found in the UP-C and UP-A in your practice and meets the needs of a wide array of client presentations and contexts. In the meantime, we recognize that there are still many goals to be achieved with our work on the UP-C and UP-A, particularly in providing clear tailoring and adaptation guidelines within the books themselves for more diverse youth samples and community settings. We realize the UP-C and UP-A itself can feel at times like a large and didactic collection of excellent behavior techniques that requires some winnowing and substantive practice to make it truly useful in the broadest range of settings and populations possible. This work is in progress and will hopefully inform a sleeker, more responsive and adaptive Unified Protocol in the future.

SUGGESTIONS FOR USING THIS VOLUME

This volume is best used alongside, rather than as a replacement for, Ehrenreich-May et al.'s (2018) *Unified Protocol for Transdiagnostic Treatment of Emotional Disorders in Children and Adolescents: Therapist Guide* and associated workbooks. The therapist guide provides a detailed introduction to each treatment and a module-by-module and/or session-by-session approach to delivering the complete set of core intervention strategies contained within the UP-C and UP-A. The therapist guide also includes detailed descriptions of activities designed to facilitate illustration and practice of core intervention components, sample scripts for therapists to utilize when introducing intervention components, helpful clinician tips, and a variety of other materials. The *Unified Protocol for Transdiagnostic Treatment of Emotional Disorders in Children: Workbook* (Ehrenreich-May et al., 2018) and *Unified Protocol for Transdiagnostic Treatment of Emotional Disorders in Adolescents: Workbook* (Ehrenreich-May et al., 2018) provide the complete set of worksheets, forms, and figures referenced in the therapist guide in two separate volumes, one for children and parents and the other for adolescents. While

Chapter 2 of this volume does provide a brief overview of how core intervention strategies in the therapist guide and workbooks are typically delivered to youth with anxiety and/or depressive disorders, this discussion is not comprehensive enough for clinicians unfamiliar with the UP-C and UP-A. Therefore, we would suggest that clinicians interested in adapting these interventions first consult and familiarize themselves with the UP-C and UP-A therapist guide and workbook materials before approaching some of the applications described in this volume. It may also be helpful for clinicians relatively new to the UP-C and/or UP-A to gain experience with delivering these interventions to several youth with more "straightforward" symptom presentations characterized primarily by anxiety or depression before attempting to adapt the interventions, although this is certainly not a requirement.

Each of the chapters in this volume describes how the content, format, and supporting materials of the UP-C and/or UP-A may need to be adapted to enhance their relevance and clinical appropriateness for the population or setting described in the chapter. To fully appreciate and contextualize these adaptations, it may be helpful for clinicians to consult the UP-C and UP-A therapist guide and workbooks as they are reading particular chapters to reference particular intervention strategies, forms, or worksheets. Each of the chapters in this volume also provides a brief case example to illustrate how to apply the adapted intervention to the clinical presentation or in the particular setting being discussed. Additionally, "tip sheets" at the end of each chapter summarize key adaptations and potential treatment barriers; we hope that these tip sheets may provide quick guides for busy clinicians who may wish to remind themselves of key points to recall about applying the UP-C and/or UP-A prior to their sessions. We have designed the format and materials in this volume with the practicing clinician in mind and hope that these tools will approachable, thorough, and user-friendly enough to facilitate more widespread use of these interventions in a variety of clinical settings.

REFERENCES

American Psychiatric Association. (2013). *Diagnostic and statistical manual of mental disorders* (5th ed.).

Angold, A., Costello, E. J., & Erkanli, A. (1999). Comorbidity. *Journal of Child Psychology and Psychiatry, 40*(1), 57–87.

Axelson, D. A., & Birmaher, B. (2001). Relation between anxiety and depressive disorders in childhood and adolescence. *Depression and Anxiety, 14*(2), 67–78.

Bardeen, J. R., Fergus, T. A., & Orcutt, H. K. (2013). Experiential avoidance as a moderator of the relationship between anxiety sensitivity and perceived stress. *Behavior Therapy, 44*(3), 459–469.

Bar-Haim, Y., Lamy, D., Pergamin, L., Bakermans-Kranenburg, M. J., & Van Ijzendoorn, M. H. (2007). Threat-related attentional bias in anxious and nonanxious individuals: A meta-analytic study. *Psychological Bulletin, 133*(1), 1–24.

Bariola, E., Hughes, E. K., & Gullone, E. (2012). Relationships between parent and child emotion regulation strategy use: A brief report. *Journal of Child and Family Studies, 21*(3), 443–448.

Barlow, D. H., Allen, L. B., & Choate, M. L. (2004). Toward a unified treatment for emotional disorders. *Behavior Therapy, 35*(2), 205–230.

Barlow, D. H., Farchione, T. J., Fairholme, C. P., Ellard, K. K., Boisseau, C. L., Allen, L. B., & Ehrenreich-May, J. (2011). *Unified protocol for transdiagnostic treatment of emotional disorders: Therapist guide*. Oxford University Press.

Benjamin, C. L., Puleo, C. M., Settipani, C. A., Brodman, D. M., Edmunds, J. M., Cummings, C. M., & Kendall, P. C. (2011). History of cognitive-behavioral therapy in youth. *Child and Adolescent Psychiatric Clinics, 20*(2), 179–189.

Campbell-Sills, L., & Barlow, D. H. (2007). Incorporating emotion regulation into conceptualizations and treatments of anxiety and mood disorders. In J. J. Gross (Ed.), *Handbook of emotion regulation* (pp. 542–559). The Guilford Press.

Cannon, M. F., & Weems, C. F. (2010). Cognitive biases in childhood anxiety disorders: Do interpretive and judgment biases distinguish anxious youth from their non-anxious peers? *Journal of Anxiety Disorders, 24*(7), 751–758.

Carthy, T., Horesh, N., Apter, A., Edge, M. D., & Gross, J. J. (2010). Emotional reactivity and cognitive regulation in anxious children. *Behaviour Research and Therapy, 48*(5), 384–393.

Chorpita, B. F., Daleiden, E. L., & Weisz, J. R. (2005). Identifying and selecting the common elements of evidence based interventions: A distillation and matching model. *Mental Health Services Research, 7*(1), 5–20.

Chorpita, B. F., Plummer, C. M., & Moffitt, C. E. (2000). Relations of tripartite dimensions of emotion to childhood anxiety and mood disorders. *Journal of Abnormal Child Psychology, 28*(3), 299–310.

Chorpita, B. F., Weisz, J. R., Daleiden, E. L., Schoenwald, S. K., Palinkas, L. A., Miranda, J., Higa-McMillan, C. K., Nakamura, B., Aukahi Austin, A., Borntrager, C. F., Ward, A., Wells, K. C., & Gibbons, R. D. (2013). Long-term outcomes for the Child STEPs randomized effectiveness trial: A comparison of modular and standard treatment designs with usual care. *Journal of Consulting and Clinical Psychology, 81*(6), 999–1009.

Chu, B. C., Colognori, D., Weissman, A. S., & Bannon, K. (2009). An initial description and pilot of group behavioral activation therapy for anxious and depressed youth. *Cognitive and Behavioral Practice, 16*(4), 408–419.

Chu, B. C., & Harrison, T. L. (2007). Disorder-specific effects of CBT for anxious and depressed youth: A meta-analysis of candidate mediators of change. *Clinical Child and Family Psychology Review, 10*(4), 352–372.

Clark, L. A., & Watson, D. (1991). Tripartite model of anxiety and depression: Psychometric evidence and taxonomic implications. *Journal of Abnormal Psychology, 100*(3), 316–336.

Cummings, J. R., Bornovalova, M. A., Ojanen, T., Hunt, E., MacPherson, L., & Lejuez, C. (2013). Time doesn't change everything: The longitudinal course of distress tolerance and its relationship with externalizing and internalizing symptoms during early adolescence. *Journal of Abnormal Child Psychology, 41*(5), 735–748.

Drake, K. L., & Ginsburg, G. S. (2012). Family factors in the development, treatment, and prevention of childhood anxiety disorders. *Clinical Child and Family Psychology Review, 15*(2), 144–162.

Ehrenreich, J. T., Goldstein, C. R., Wright, L. R., & Barlow, D. H. (2009). Development of a unified protocol for the treatment of emotional disorders in youth. *Child & Family Behavior Therapy, 31*(1), 20–37.

Ehrenreich-May, J., & Bilek, E. L. (2012). The development of a transdiagnostic, cognitive behavioral group intervention for childhood anxiety disorders and co-occurring depression symptoms. *Cognitive and Behavioral Practice, 19*(1), 41–55.

Ehrenreich-May, J., Kennedy, S. M., Sherman, J. A., Bennett, S. M., & Barlow, D. H. (2018). *Unified protocol for transdiagnostic treatment of emotional disorders in adolescents: Workbook.* Oxford University Press.

Ehrenreich-May, J., Kennedy, S. M., Sherman, J. A., Bilek, E. L., & Barlow, D. H. (2018). *Unified protocol for transdiagnostic treatment of emotional disorders in children: Workbook.* Oxford University Press.

Ehrenreich-May, J., Kennedy, S. M., Sherman, J. A., Bilek, E. L., Buzzella, B. A., Bennett, S. M., & Barlow, D. H. (2017). *Unified protocols for transdiagnostic treatment of emotional disorders in children and adolescents: Therapist guide.* Oxford University Press.

Garber, J., & Weersing, V. R. (2010). Comorbidity of anxiety and depression in youth: Implications for treatment and prevention. *Clinical Psychology: Science and Practice, 17*(4), 293–306.

Gross, J. J., & Thompson, R. A. (2007). Emotion regulation: Conceptual foundations. In J. J. Gross (Ed.), *Handbook of emotion regulation* (p. 3-24).Guilford Press.

Hankin, B. L. (2008). Rumination and depression in adolescence: Investigating symptom specificity in a multiwave prospective study. *Journal of Clinical Child & Adolescent Psychology, 37*(4), 701–713.

Kendall, P. C. (1994). Treating anxiety disorders in children: Results of a randomized clinical trial. *Journal of Consulting and Clinical Psychology, 62*(1), 100.

Kennedy, S. M., Tonarely, N. A., Halliday, E., & Ehrenreich-May, J. (Under Review). A person-centered approach to understanding heterogeneity of youth receiving transdiagnostic treatment for emotional disorders.

Laurent, J., Catanzaro, S. J., & Joiner Jr, T. E. (2004). Development and preliminary validation of the Physiological Hyperarousal Scale for Children. *Psychological Assessment, 16*(4), 373–380.

Marchette, L. K., & Weisz, J. R. (2017). Practitioner review: Empirical evolution of youth psychotherapy toward transdiagnostic approaches. *Journal of Child Psychology and Psychiatry, 58*(9), 970–984.

Martinsen, K. D., Kendall, P. C., Stark, K., & Neumer, S. P. (2016). Prevention of anxiety and depression in children: Acceptability and feasibility of the transdiagnostic EMOTION program. *Cognitive and Behavioral Practice, 23*(1), 1–13.

McHugh, R. K., Reynolds, E. K., Leyro, T. M., & Otto, M. W. (2013). An examination of the association of distress intolerance and emotion regulation with avoidance. *Cognitive Therapy and Research, 37*(2), 363–367.

McLaughlin, K. A., & Nolen-Hoeksema, S. (2011). Rumination as a transdiagnostic factor in depression and anxiety. *Behaviour Research and Therapy, 49*(3), 186–193.

Ollendick, T. H., Jarrett, M. A., Grills-Taquechel, A. E., Hovey, L. D., & Wolff, J. C. (2008). Comorbidity as a predictor and moderator of treatment outcome in youth with anxiety, affective, attention deficit/hyperactivity disorder, and oppositional/conduct disorders. *Clinical Psychology Review, 28*(8), 1447–1471.

Patterson, G. R. (1982). *Coercive family process* (Vol. 3). Castalia Publishing Company.

Platt, B., Waters, A. M., Schulte-Koerne, G., Engelmann, L., & Salemink, E. (2017). A review of cognitive biases in youth depression: Attention, interpretation and memory. *Cognition and Emotion, 31*(3), 462–483.

Rogers, M. L., Halberstadt, A. G., Castro, V. L., MacCormack, J. K., & Garrett-Peters, P. (2016). Maternal emotion socialization differentially predicts third-grade children's emotion regulation and lability. *Emotion, 16*(2), 280–291.

Suveg, C., Hudson, J. L., Brewer, G., Flannery-Schroeder, E., Gosch, E., & Kendall, P. C. (2009). Cognitive-behavioral therapy for anxiety-disordered youth: Secondary outcomes from a randomized clinical trial evaluating child and family modalities. *Journal of Anxiety Disorders, 23*(3), 341–349.

Thompson-Hollands, J., Kerns, C. E., Pincus, D. B., & Comer, J. S. (2014). Parental accommodation of child anxiety and related symptoms: Range, impact, and correlates. *Journal of Anxiety Disorders, 28*(8), 765–773.

Weisz, J., Bearman, S. K., Santucci, L. C., & Jensen-Doss, A. (2017). Initial test of a principle-guided approach to transdiagnostic psychotherapy with children and adolescents. *Journal of Clinical Child & Adolescent Psychology, 46*(1), 44–58.

Weisz, J. R., Chorpita, B. F., Palinkas, L. A., Schoenwald, S. K., Miranda, J., Bearman, S. K., Daleiden, E. L., Ugueto, A. M., Ho, A., Martin, J., Gray, J., Alleyne, A., Langer, D. A., Southam-Gerow, M. A., & Gibbons, R. D. (2012). Testing standard and modular designs for psychotherapy treating depression, anxiety, and conduct problems in youth: A randomized effectiveness trial. *Archives of General Psychiatry, 69*(3), 274–282.

Weisz, J. R., McCarty, C. A., & Valeri, S. M. (2006). Effects of psychotherapy for depression in children and adolescents: A meta-analysis. *Psychological Bulletin, 132*(1), 132–149.

Wilamowska, Z. A., Thompson-Hollands, J., Fairholme, C. P., Ellard, K. K., Farchione, T. J., & Barlow, D. H. (2010). Conceptual background, development, and preliminary data from the unified protocol for transdiagnostic treatment of emotional disorders. *Depression and Anxiety, 27*(10), 882–890.

Williams, A. D., Thompson, J., & Andrews, G. (2013). The impact of psychological distress tolerance in the treatment of depression. *Behaviour Research and Therapy, 51*(8), 469–475.

Zvolensky, M. J., Vujanovic, A. A., Bernstein, A., & Leyro, T. (2010). Distress tolerance: Theory, measurement, and relations to psychopathology. *Current Directions in Psychological Science, 19*(6), 406–410.

2

Delivery of Standard UP-C and UP-A Treatment for Youth with Emotional Disorders

RINATTE GRUEN AND DYLAN BRAUN ■

The therapist manuals for the Unified Protocols for Transdiagnostic Treatment of Emotional Disorders in Children (UP-C) and Adolescents (UP-A) are presented in two halves of a joint therapist guide (Ehrenreich-May et al., 2018). While the two manuals differ in their format and developmental modifications, the UP-A and UP-C share a single set of core transdiagnostic intervention principles and can be particularly useful for youth presenting with multiple disorders and/or subclinical symptoms. The UP-A, developed for individual treatment with adolescents aged 12 to 18, includes eight modules focused on the adolescent client and a separate module (Module P) focused on caregiver skills, which can be used at the therapist's discretion. Treatment with the UP-A varies in length based on client need, although the typical course of treatment ranges from 12 to 16 sessions. The UP-C was designed to be presented in 15, 1.5-hour group therapy sessions with six- to 12-year-old children. Caregivers typically play an active role in the UP-C, attending caregiver-focused sessions and joining the children's group to practice skills together. The metaphor of Emotion Detectives is used throughout the UP-C, with children learning to "solve the mystery of emotions" and acquiring CLUES skills (Consider How I Feel, Look at My Thoughts, Use Detective Thinking and Problem Solving, Experience My Emotions, and Stay Healthy and Happy) over the course of treatment. While the UP-A was developed for individual treatment and the UP-C was designed for group therapy, both treatments can be adapted for either group or individual delivery. The suggested age ranges for each treatment noted earlier should serve as a general guideline, and therapists should use clinical judgment to determine the developmentally appropriate manual to use with each client.

This chapter describes the core components and associated treatment skills that cut across the UP-C and UP-A, including their placement and presentation in the UP-C and UP-A therapist guide. As such, this chapter may provide a refresher for clinicians returning to the UP-C/A after some time, and it can be a helpful summary for those who are newer to the protocols. Throughout the descriptions of the various modules, the chapter will compare and contrast how the core treatment components are presented in the UP-C and UP-A. Although this chapter focuses on how UP-C/A treatment components can be utilized to address anxiety and depression concerns in youth, it also provides context for the adaptations for other symptom areas that are described later in the book. For easy reference, Table 2.1 presents the UP-A core components by module, while Table 2.2 presents the UP-C core components by module and CLUES skill. Table 2.3 lists key differences in the typical delivery of UP-C and UP-A materials.

UP-A MODULE 1/UP-C SESSION 1: BUILDING MOTIVATION AND IDENTIFYING TREATMENT GOALS

The beginning of treatment focuses on building rapport, enhancing motivation, identifying treatment goals, and addressing obstacles to care. This content area generally is covered in the first one or two sessions of UP-A or the first session of UP-C. From the outset, therapists should set the tone for treatment by emphasizing that the purpose of the UP-A or UP-C is *not* to eliminate emotions, but rather to learn strategies to reduce distress caused by emotional experiences and to learn new, more helpful ways of acting in response to emotions.

In the UP-A, therapists develop rapport through one-on-one conversations and activities with their clients, during which time therapists may learn about the clients' experiences and their perspectives on treatment. The therapist guide (Ehrenreich-May et al., 2018) provides a brief introduction to motivational interviewing techniques, and therapists may devote a second session to additional rapport building and motivational enhancement for reluctant clients. The UP-C utilizes fun activities, crafts, and team-building exercises to help build positive relationships between clients, therapists, and families participating in the group. During the first session, children decorate small containers that serve as CLUES kits, in which they store reward tokens that they earn for engaging in sessions and completing home learning assignments. This fun activity serves a rapport-building function and also sets the stage for the therapists to use frequent reinforcement to build and maintain motivation throughout treatment.

Progress monitoring is an important component of the UP-A and UP-C. Through interactive discussion, therapists work with their clients to develop a list of three or more Top Problems (Weisz et al., 2011), key areas in which the youth engage in unhelpful emotional behaviors in response to strong emotions. Top Problems reflect areas of focus for treatment and can be helpful in personalizing intervention delivery. During each session, the client and parent rate the level of impairment associated with each Top Problem. In the UP-A, adolescents and

Table 2.1 UP-A CORE COMPONENTS BY MODULE

Module	Title	Recommended # of Sessions	Core Components
1	Building and Keeping Motivation	1–2	• Identification of problems and goals • Enhancing motivation for change
2	Getting to Know Your Emotions and Behaviors	2–3	• Enhancing emotional awareness • Connecting emotional responses to behaviors
3	Introduction to Emotion-Focused Behavioral Experiments	1–2	• Modifying behavioral action tendencies
4	Awareness of Physical Sensations	1–2	• Increasing awareness and tolerance of physical sensations
5	Being Flexible in Your Thinking	2–3	• Promoting cognitive flexibility through detective thinking and problem solving
6	Awareness of Emotional Experiences	1–2	• Increasing awareness and tolerance of emotional experiences
7	Situational Emotion Exposure	2+	• Reducing avoidance and modifying behavioral action tendencies
8	Reviewing Accomplishments and Looking Ahead	1	• Maintaining gains and preventing relapse
P	Parenting the Emotional Adolescent	1–3	• Increasing consistency • Reducing accommodation • Replacing criticism with empathy and positive reinforcement • Modeling healthy and helpful emotional responses

their parents often initially are asked to develop Top Problems separately, with the therapist working later in session to help consolidate these lists. If there is strong disagreement, the adolescent and their parent can each rate their own list of Top Problems over the course of treatment. In the UP-C group, Top Problems most often are generated at the beginning of the initial session through collaboration among the child, parent, and therapist. In the UP-C/A, therapists work with their clients to develop SMART (Specific, Measurable, Attainable, Relevant, and

Table 2.2 UP-C CHILD AND PARENT CORE COMPONENTS BY SESSION

CLUES (Emotion Detective) Skills	Session	Child Core Components	Parent Core Components
"C" Skill (Consider How I Feel)	UP-C Session 1: Introduction to the UP-C Treatment Model	• Identification of problems and goals • Enhancing emotional awareness	• Enhancing motivation • Promoting parent awareness of child emotional responding
	UP-C Session 2: Getting to Know Your Emotions	• Enhancing emotional awareness • Connecting emotional responses to behaviors	• Connecting child emotional responding to parent emotional responding • Encouraging positive reinforcement as an opposite parenting behavior to criticism
	UP-C Session 3: Using Science Experiments to Change Our Emotions and Behavior	• Modifying behavioral action tendencies	• Encouraging positive reinforcement as an opposite parenting behavior to criticism
	UP-C Session 4: Our Body Clues	• Increasing awareness and tolerance of physical sensations	• Increasing parent awareness and tolerance of physical sensations • Encouraging empathy as an opposite parenting behavior to criticism
"L" Skill (Look at My Thoughts)	UP-C Session 5: Look at My Thoughts	• Promoting cognitive flexibility by increasing awareness of thinking traps	• Promoting consistent reinforcement and discipline
"U" Skill (Use Detective Thinking and Problem Solving)	UP-C Session 6: Use Detective Thinking	• Promoting cognitive flexibility through detective thinking	• Increasing parent cognitive flexibility • Replacing accommodation with healthy independence granting
	UP-C Session 7: Problem Solving and Conflict Management	• Promoting cognitive flexibility through problem solving	• Replacing accommodation with healthy independence granting

"E" Skill (Experience My Emotions)

UP-C **Session 8:** Awareness of Emotional Experiences

UP-C **Session 9:** Introduction to Emotion Exposure

- Increasing awareness and tolerance of emotional experiences
- Reducing avoidance and modifying behavioral action tendencies

- Increasing parent awareness and tolerance of emotional experiences
- Planning for situational emotion exposure
- Promoting healthy and helpful parent modeling of emotions
- Planning for situational emotion exposure
- Using opposite parenting behaviors to support exposures

UP-C **Session 10:** Facing Our Feelings—Part 1

- Reducing avoidance and modifying behavioral action tendencies

UP-C **Sessions 11-14:** Facing Our Feelings—Part 2

- Reducing avoidance and modifying behavioral action tendencies

- Parent incorporation in situational emotion exposures as indicated

UP-C **Session 15:** Wrap-Up and Relapse Prevention

- Maintaining gains and preventing relapse

- Maintaining gains and preventing relapse

"S" Skill (Stay Healthy and Happy)

Table 2.3 KEY DIFFERENCES IN HOW TREATMENT COMPONENTS ARE PRESENTED
IN UP-A AND UP-C

Treatment Component	UP-A	UP-C
Motivational Enhancement (UP-A Module 1/UP-C Session 1)	Individual rapport building and motivational interviewing (as needed)	Group rapport building and motivational enhancement through fun activities and team-building exercises. A token-economy system can reinforce engagement in sessions.
Emotion Identification (UP-A Module 2/UP-C Sessions 1–2)	Guided discussion of commonly experienced emotions, utilizing worksheets as aids	Greater emphasis is placed on helping children understand the gradient of emotion intensity, using interactive tools like a large-scale emotion thermometer.
Opposite Action (UP-A Module 3/UP-C Session 3)	Use of "science experiment" language to introduce opposite actions is optional. Adolescents are asked to engage in more intensive tracking of opposite actions and their impact on emotions for home learning.	Therapists are encouraged to use the language of a "science experiment" when introducing opposite actions. Children engage in opposite action in session (e.g., by engaging in a dance party or other physical activity in session) and monitor changes to their emotions.
Body Clues (UP-A Module 4/UP-C Session 4)	Therapists encourage adolescents to identify their physical sensations associated with strong emotions using a worksheet depicting the outline of a body. Sensational exposures can be more personalized in the individual therapy setting.	Discussion of body clues is similar to that in the UP-A, although children may benefit from creating life-sized body outlines to identify physical sensations.
Thinking Traps and Detective Thinking (UP-A Module 5/UP-C Sessions 5–7)	Adolescents are introduced to a more extensive list of thinking traps and detective questions they may wish to use to generate evidence when evaluating thinking traps.	Children are introduced to only four common thinking traps, using memorable thinking trap characters (e.g., "Jumping Jack" for "Jumping to Conclusions"). Additionally, children engage in a detective activity in which they are tasked to collect clues to solve a non-emotional "mystery" before learning to apply these steps to their own thinking traps. Detective thinking steps are referred to as the "Stop, Slow, Go" steps to promote retention.

Table 2.3 CONTINUED

Treatment Component	UP-A	UP-C
Mindfulness/ Awareness (UP-A Module 6/UP-C Session 8)	Present moment awareness and nonjudgmental awareness are presented through activities and role plays. Generalized emotion exposures are introduced to promote present-moment and non-judgmental awareness to emotional experiences in session.	Present-moment awareness activities are more concrete and make greater use of the five senses (e.g., "Five Senses Game"). Nonjudgmental awareness is simplified. Generalized emotion exposures are not introduced in this session, although they can be incorporated into situational exposures.
Exposures (UP-A Module 7/UP-C Sessions 9–14)	The purpose of exposure is introduced to adolescents using emotion curves depicting the typical changes in emotional intensity during escape/ avoidance behaviors, habituation, and practice over time.	• Although emotion curves may be used in UP-C, exposures are generally introduced through therapist modeling with a stuffed animal or other toy. In the group setting, children complete a group-based exposure before moving on to individual exposures. • Although UP-A therapists may choose to have a parent-focused session at this point in treatment, more direct guidance is given in the UP-C to help parents support their children in planning and completing exposures.
Wrap-Up/Relapse Prevention (UP-A Module 8/UP-C Session 15)	Adolescents are given opportunities to reflect on and celebrate their treatment accomplishments through discussion with their therapist and review of Top Problem data.	Therapists generally have a party with the children to celebrate their accomplishments during treatment, and the puzzle pieces collected throughout the course of treatment are assembled as a group to reveal an associated prize (e.g., a special snack, party decorations).

Time-bound) goals associated with each Top Problem to promote motivation for engagement. Progress toward these goals can serve as indicators of change over the course of therapy.

During the first session, therapists also work with clients and parents to identify potential barriers to treatment attendance or engagement. If needed, the therapist may use problem-solving techniques to generate solutions to these obstacles to care.

UP-A MODULE 2/UP-C SESSIONS 1 AND 2: IDENTIFYING EMOTIONS AND EMOTIONAL BEHAVIORS

The second set of core treatment skills focuses on psychoeducation about the purpose of emotions, the three-component model of emotions, and the cycle of avoidance. This content area is presented in the second module of the UP-A, which is covered over the course of two or three sessions. In the UP-C group, this material spans the first and second sessions and begins the Consider How I Feel skill, which extends through the fourth session. Key to the discussion of emotions across both the UP-C and UP-A is the concept that emotions are "normal, natural, and harmless." In the UP-A, therapists can flexibly use a simple worksheet listing different emotion words to assess aspects of adolescents' emotional awareness (e.g., emotion vocabulary, emotional clarity), as well as those emotions adolescents experience most and least often. In the UP-C, therapists promote emotional awareness through group didactic instruction and through an interactive emotion thermometer activity designed to enhance emotional vocabulary and promote understanding of emotional gradient. Children participating in the UP-C also play an alarm game, in which they differentiate "true alarms" (truly threatening situations) from "false alarms" (situations that *feel* threatening but are not actually dangerous). In both treatment protocols, the therapist introduces youths to the idea of emotional behaviors, which are behaviors motivated by emotional experiences. These behaviors can be helpful (e.g., moving out of the way of a speeding car due to fear) or maladaptive (e.g., avoiding participating in class due to anxiety).

In both the UP-C and UP-A, an additional key component of this content area is teaching clients to break down their emotional experiences and understand the connection between their thoughts, physical sensations ("body clues" in UP-C), and behaviors. Although it is helpful for clients to practice breaking down personal examples of intense emotional experiences, this process can be scaffolded by progressing from hypothetical examples, to lower-intensity personally salient examples, and then to more intense emotional experiences. In both the UP-A and UP-C, therapists and their clients discuss the cycle of avoidance and other emotional behaviors. Clients begin tracking their emotional experience using the "Tracking the Before, During, and After." (BDA) functional assessment tool, which parses the antecedents, responses, and short- and long-term consequences of their reactions to emotional experiences.

UP-A MODULE 3/UP-C SESSION 3: INTRODUCTION TO EMOTION-FOCUSED BEHAVIORAL EXPERIMENTS

Module 3 of the UP-A and the third session of the UP-C introduce the core treatment skills of acting opposite to emotionally driven behaviors and the use of emotion-focused behavioral experiments. In the UP-C and UP-A, "acting opposite" refers to engaging in an action counter to a person's predominant (maladaptive) response to strong emotions. For example, instead of procrastinating on an assignment due to fear of not completing it perfectly (i.e., an emotionally driven avoidance behavior), an opposite action might be to begin working on a small part of the assignment immediately after getting home from school (i.e., an approach-oriented behavior). Clients practice acting opposite in the context of emotion-focused behavioral experiments (described to children as "science experiments" in the UP-C). These experiments serve as information-gathering exercises, in that clients are asked to test out hypotheses about how acting opposite to an emotional behavior might impact their emotional experience.

In standard applications of the UP-C/A, therapists guide youth through a series of activities to help them practice acting opposite to predominant action urges for sadness (e.g., withdrawal, isolation, engaging in low-energy activities) during and outside of session. The therapist might introduce this concept by asking the child or adolescent to dance to an upbeat song in session and to notice the impact of this action on their emotion level. Therapists enhance the client's understanding of the connection between emotion and activity by introducing a sample emotion and activity diary and teaching the client to track their emotion and activity levels throughout the week. Clients work with the therapist to create a list of enjoyable or valued activities and plan times throughout the week to engage in these activities when they might experience a strong emotion. Of note, while standard UP-C and UP-A applications focus on "acting opposite" to sadness in this session, the activity list and home learning assignments for this session can easily be tailored to reinforce acting opposite practice for a variety of strong emotions.

UP-A MODULE 4/UP-C SESSION 4: AWARENESS OF PHYSICAL SENSATIONS

Awareness of physical sensations and their connection to strong emotions encompasses the fourth core skill in UP-A and UP-C. Clinicians cover this material during one or two sessions in the fourth module of the UP-A, and in the fourth session of the UP-C. Additional psychoeducation about physical sensations or "body clues" (e.g., fight or flight) is provided to normalize the physiological component of emotions and correct unhelpful beliefs about physical sensations. Clients then engage in several activities to promote identification and awareness of physical sensations. Clients use a body outline or tracings of their own body (in UP-C) to identify the location of physical sensations in their body for different strong emotions. To promote awareness of physical sensations and prevent unhelpful cognitive and behavioral responses to body sensations, clients are introduced to body scanning, a skill that helps youth stay in the present moment while experiencing uncomfortable body sensations (that are not indicative of actual threat). In the UP-C/A, clinicians promote the use of mindfulness techniques during these sensational exposures, providing a chance for young clients to build greater awareness of the somatic component of their emotional experiences. While interoceptive exposures are known to be especially beneficial for youth with panic symptoms or strong anxiety sensitivity, the UP-C/A emphasizes that they can be successfully utilized with a wide range of clients with somatic symptoms to reduce distress associated with these symptoms. During sensational exposures such as running in place or breathing through a straw, therapists encourage their clients to use body-scanning techniques to notice physical sensations, rate the intensity of these sensations, and watch as the sensations abate naturally over time. Through these activities, clients learn that physical sensations—while uncomfortable—are not actually dangerous and do not need to be alleviated through engaging in emotional behaviors.

UP-A MODULE 5/UP-C SESSIONS 5 TO 7: FLEXIBLE THINKING

Enhancing cognitive flexibility and linking thoughts to emotions, both in and before entering emotional situations, is the fifth core skill in UP-C and UP-A. In the UP-A, this core skill is covered in Module 5, which is typically delivered in two or three sessions. In the UP-C, components designed to increase cognitive flexibility fall under the umbrella of Look at My Thoughts ("L" of the CLUES skills) and Use Detective Thinking and Problem Solving ("U" of the CLUES skills) during the fifth, sixth, and seventh sessions of treatment. Youth with emotional disorders often develop unhelpful patterns of thinking ("cognitive biases") that increase negative emotionality and maintain unhelpful cycles of avoidance and other emotional behaviors. Treatment components focused on flexible thinking teach youth to recognize unhelpful automatic interpretations and practice cognitive reappraisal to challenge those interpretations. Youth also are taught problem solving as a means of addressing daily life challenges, including interpersonal difficulties, with flexibility.

Clinicians introduce the concept of automatic thoughts (termed "snap judgments" in the UP-C) through engaging youth in a discussion of competing possible interpretations of a series of ambiguous images (e.g., the "old lady/young lady" picture). Discussion of these ambiguous images yields observations that we often become "locked into" our first interpretation of a situation, making it difficult to see other possibilities, even though this initial interpretation may not always be the most helpful or realistic. "Thinking traps" are then introduced in the UP-C/A as types of automatic thoughts or snap judgments; strong emotions can increase youth susceptibility to thinking traps, and thinking traps can increase the frequency and intensity of strong emotions. Presentation of thinking traps in the UP-C and UP-A is developmentally tailored in several notable ways. Children are introduced to four thinking traps in the UP-C (in contrast to upwards of 10 in the UP-A), and appealing and memorable characters are assigned to each UP-C thinking trap to improve engagement and retention of material. Accordingly, while the cognitive distortion of "Probability Estimation" is introduced in the UP-A as "Jumping to Conclusions," this thinking trap is linked in the UP-C to the memorable character of "Jumping Jack," who is almost certain that there is a high likelihood his plane will crash. After being asked to generate examples of and track their own personal thinking traps, youth are taught "detective thinking" (i.e., cognitive restructuring) in both the UP-C and UP-A to learn to question and critically evaluate their automatic thoughts. Crucially, the goal of detective thinking is to learn to think *flexibly* rather than positively or even accurately, and to learn to generate more helpful alternative thoughts that may be applied to future situations. As an extension of cognitive flexibility, youth learn a series of problem-solving steps to enhance their ability to think flexibly about potential solutions to problems they typically encounter in daily life, particularly in their interpersonal relationships. Clinicians emphasize the importance of learning to use detective thinking and problem solving *before* entering into emotional situations, as high levels of emotional arousal can interfere with cognitive processing and reinstate rigid patterns of thinking and responding.

UP-A MODULE 6, UP-C SESSION 8: PRESENT-MOMENT AND NONJUDGMENTAL AWARENESS

The sixth core skill in the UP-C and UP-A involves enhancing awareness of emotional experiences through present-moment awareness or mindfulness techniques. In the UP-A, this skill is presented in Module 6, typically over one or two sessions. In the UP-C, this skill is delivered in Session 8 as a part of Experience My Emotions ("E" of the CLUES skills). This material builds on previously introduced skills, including the body-scanning technique from UP-A Module 4 and UP-C Session 4 that youth learned to practice as a means of "sticking with" their uncomfortable body sensations. When introducing youth to present-moment awareness, it can be useful for clinicians to consider its utility as a form of opposite action to cognitive avoidance techniques like distraction and thought suppression, as well as to other emotional behaviors like rumination. Whereas the cognitive flexibility skills introduced in the previous section are best practiced before entering emotional situations, present-moment awareness techniques can be practiced before, during, and after emotional experiences.

Especially for younger children, or youth who may be particularly avoidant of their emotional experiences, it is helpful for clinicians to begin by introducing the rationale for fully experiencing emotions by using awareness techniques. Present-moment awareness can then be introduced as the practice of noticing, describing, and experiencing aspects of the present moment, including the youth's surroundings, emotional experiences, and/or interactions. In the UP-C, children gradually progress to practicing awareness of emotional experiences through the "My Five Senses Game," during which they are first asked to practice awareness of non-emotional experiences through several interactive exercises. Nonjudgmental awareness is then presented to youth as a compassionate, accepting form of awareness of their emotional experiences. As with other UP-C and UP-A skills, nonjudgmental awareness may be introduced using impersonal and non-emotional examples, such as by asking youth to practice describing everyday objects without judgments. For youth who struggle to adopt a nonjudgmental attitude toward their own emotions, clinicians can illustrate this skill by having youth role play a conversation between themselves and a self-critical friend, encouraging clients to show compassion to themselves as they would to a friend. In the UP-A, these mindful awareness skills are practiced further through generalized emotion exposures. Clients may be asked to write about an emotional experience or to engage with an emotionally evocative song or video while practicing nonjudgmental present-moment awareness, rather than avoiding or distracting from these experiences or suppressing their emotional responses.

UP-C MODULE 7, UP-A SESSIONS 9 TO 14: EXPOSURES AND EMOTION-FOCUSED BEHAVIORAL EXPERIMENTS

The second-to-last and typically the longest section of the UP-C/A primarily focuses on situational exposure, a core component of many cognitive-behavioral interventions. While most often associated with anxiety-focused interventions, exposures in the UP-C and UP-A are practiced as a means of reducing emotional responding, increasing distress tolerance, and disconfirming inaccurate or unhelpful cognitions related to any emotion-related trigger. The seventh module of the UP-A is completed over at least two sessions, and the number of sessions spent on this module varies depending on the needs of the client. If a client has already demonstrated a treatment response prior to this module, it is still recommended that they be guided through at least a few situational exposures, both due to their potential importance for extending and maintaining treatment gains and so the client can continue to implement this skill on their own after treatment. Within the UP-C, clients practice exposures in the Experience My Emotions section of treatment, spanning the ninth through 14th sessions. Exposure practice should continue until the client has experienced significant treatment response and/or is ready to continue exposure efforts without the therapist's weekly support.

After briefly reviewing skills learned in earlier sections of treatment, the therapist presents the rationale for exposure and connects this technique to other emotion-focused experiments, such as opposite action and interoceptive exposure. Clients and their parents then work to develop a list of situations in which they currently engage in unhelpful emotional behaviors like avoidance, rumination, or reassurance seeking. Guided by their therapists, youth practice entering into these challenging situations without relying on their emotional behaviors. As an alternative, they are reminded of the appropriate times to utilize various UP-C/A skills, including detective thinking, present-moment awareness, and nonjudgmental awareness. As youth attempt increasingly difficult exposures, their emotional responsiveness to these situations often reduces and their confidence in their ability to tolerate distress without engaging in safety or avoidance behaviors improves. Safety learning also occurs, such that youth begin to recognize that the probability of a negative outcome occurring is much lower than they originally believed, and the occurrence of a negative outcome is generally not catastrophic.

Consistent exposure practice both in session and for home learning is crucial for youth to make consistent progress and for gains to generalize across situations. As an optional therapy goal, therapists can modify exposures to meet additional treatment targets, such as helping the client develop stronger social skills or adding response-prevention steps for youth with compulsive behaviors. The overarching goal here is to adapt exposure efforts to increase the overall benefits to the client. Common adaptations will be discussed in subsequent chapters of this guide.

UP-A MODULE 8, UP-C SESSION 15: REVIEWING ACCOMPLISHMENTS AND LOOKING AHEAD

Module 8 of the UP-A and Session 15 of the UP-C (Stay Healthy and Happy, or the "S" CLUES skill) represent the final session of treatment. This session consists of skills review, celebration of progress, and planning for the future. Clients and parents are engaged in skills review and are encouraged to develop a plan for sustaining progress on treatment goals after termination. Clinicians also facilitate conversations to help clients and families distinguish between a temporary worsening of symptoms (lapse) and a more impairing return of symptom (relapse) indicative of a need to pursue further treatment. This session also provides an opportunity to discuss changes in Top Problem ratings over the course of therapy, allowing for a data-driven evaluation of treatment progress. Youth and their families are encouraged to reflect on their respective accomplishments, noting improvements in their ability to manage strong emotions. In the UP-C, children and their families have a chance to celebrate the progress they made as a group, and this final group session can have the atmosphere of a graduation party.

PARENT-FOCUSED CONTENT

Parent engagement is considered a critical component of both the UP-C and the UP-A; consistent with the changing role parents play in supporting skills acquisition and emotion regulation across development, the UP-C includes a structured parent component in almost every group session, while UP-A parenting materials can be applied more flexibly on an as-indicated basis. While parents are typically involved in discussion of Top Problem ratings and review of child-focused skills in nearly every session, the therapist guide provides a separate parent-focused curriculum in both the UP-C and UP-A that teaches parents to identify their "emotional parenting behaviors" and shift to using "opposite parenting behaviors," with the goal of helping children respond more adaptively to their strong emotions. Just as the early stages of UP-C and UP-A focus on promoting youth emotional awareness, the parent curriculum promotes parent awareness of both their child's emotional experience and their own emotional responses through introduction of the "Double Before, During, After" (Double BDA) exercise. This exercise helps parents build awareness of the ways in which their responses to the youth's strong emotions may decrease, maintain, or intensify the youth's emotional response. Emotional parenting behaviors are then introduced as parenting behaviors supported by research to be *less helpful* responses to youth emotional distress and include (1) overcontrol and overprotection, (2) criticism, (3) inconsistency, and (4) excessive modeling of intense emotions and avoidance. The UP-C/A pairs these unhelpful parenting behaviors with the opposite parenting strategies of (1) granting healthy independence, (2) expressing empathy and using positive reinforcement, (3) consistent use of discipline and praise, and (4) healthy emotional modeling. In contrast to emotional parenting behaviors that may serve to reinforce—or escalate—children's maladaptive reactions to strong emotions, these positive parenting techniques can promote children's ability to cope with challenging situations and react adaptively. The parenting material parallels the work done with children, encouraging families to notice maladaptive patterns, experiment with opposite actions, and learn healthy ways of responding to strong emotions.

One final and important point to note about the UP-C and UP-A is that while these treatments are presented in a sequential format, clinicians who are more experienced in these interventions may wish to rearrange, repeat, or even eliminate some modules or components, in accordance with client and setting characteristics. The UP-C and UP-A are designed to accommodate this type of flexible presentation, although evidence-based guidelines are still forthcoming.

REFERENCES

Ehrenreich-May, J., Kennedy, S. M., Sherman, J. A., Bennett, S. M., & Barlow, D. H. (2018). *Unified protocol for transdiagnostic treatment of emotional disorders in children and adolescents: Therapist guide*. Oxford University Press.

Weisz, J. R., Chorpita, B. F., Frye, A., Ng, M. Y., Lau, N., Bearman, S. K., & Hoagwood, K. E. (2011). Youth top problems: Using idiographic, consumer-guided assessment to identify treatment needs and to track change during psychotherapy. *Journal of Consulting and Clinical Psychology, 9*(3), 369–380. doi:10.1037/a0023307

3

Current Evidence Base for the UP-C and UP-A

NIZA TONARELY AND DOMINIQUE PHILLIPS ■

The Unified Protocol for Transdiagnostic Treatment of Emotional Disorders in Children and Adolescents (UP-C/A; Ehrenreich-May et al., 2018) is a core-dysfunction–based, transdiagnostic treatment for youth aged six to 18 years. The UP-C and UP-A have been adapted from the Unified Protocol for Transdiagnostic Treatment of Emotional Disorders (UP; Barlow et al., 2017b) to target emotional disorders, including anxiety, depressive, trauma-related, and obsessive-compulsive disorders, in children and adolescents. The purpose of this chapter is to review the current evidence base supporting the use of the UP-C and UP-A to treat mood and anxiety disorders in children and adolescents, respectively. We also briefly discuss the evidence base for the UP, although a more extensive discussion of this evidence base, as well as of applications of the UP to various diagnostic presentations and settings, can be found in Barlow and Farchione's (2017) *Applications of the Unified Protocol for Transdiagnostic Treatment of Emotional Disorders*, also published in the ABCT Clinical Practice Series. Research on the feasibility, acceptability, efficacy, and/or effectiveness of the UP-C and UP-A for other diagnoses and presenting concerns (e.g., obsessive-compulsive disorder, irritability, serious mental illness) will be presented in other chapters of this book.

Transdiagnostic treatments are those that aim to address a range of psychopathology and have been found to fall into three categories depending on theory: universally applied therapeutic principles, modular approaches, and shared mechanisms or core-dysfunction–based approaches (Chu, 2012; Marchette & Weisz, 2017; Sauer-Zavala et al., 2017). A universally applied therapeutic principle approach applies one set of theoretical principles to a range of diagnoses (Leichsenring & Salzer, 2014). Modular approaches allow a clinician to choose from a set of empirically derived strategies for a presenting problem, regardless of diagnosis (e.g., Chorpita & Weisz, 2009). Lastly, shared mechanisms approaches are those that target common vulnerabilities for the development and maintenance of disorders (e.g., UP; Barlow et al., 2017b). Within adult samples, transdiagnostic treatments have evidenced strong support (Barlow et al., 2004; Fairburn et al., 2003, 2009; Newby et al, 2015; Norton & Barrera, 2012; Norton & Philipp, 2008). These treatments have also shown promising results in children and adolescents (Chu et al., 2016; Harvey, 2016; Loeb et al., 2012).

The UP is one type of shared mechanisms approach to transdiagnostic treatment that was developed to target core dysfunctions across mood and anxiety disorders, previously discussed in Chapter 1 of this book (Sauer-Zavala et al., 2017). The efficacy of the UP has been investigated using open-trial formats and randomized controlled trials (RCTs), which provided support for pre- to post-UP treatment improvements in emotional disorder symptoms and negative affect from pre- to post-treatment, as well as at the six-month follow-up (Ellard et al., 2010). Compared to a waitlist control, Farchione et al. (2012) found that the UP was efficacious in reducing symptom severity and improving functional impairment. Using a randomized clinical equivalence trial, the UP was found to be as efficacious in improving anxiety symptoms as disorder-specific protocols (Barlow et al., 2017a). The UP has been extended to a range of other diagnoses and presenting concerns, including eating disorders, non-suicidal self-injury, borderline personality disorder, and bipolar disorder, among others (Bentley et al., 2017; Ellard et al., 2012; Lopez et al., 2015; Sauer-Zavala et al., 2016; Thompson-Brenner et al., 2019).

The UP-A, which was developed prior to the UP-C and in concert with the development of the adult UP, focuses on core principles similar to those found in the adult UP but delivers those principles in an adolescent-friendly format. Although there are no clear empirical guidelines for when to use the UP-A versus the UP for older adolescents and transition-age adults, therapists should consider the cognitive and developmental level of the client, the client's living situation (i.e., if the client is living with parents or other caregivers), and the impact of parenting on the client's symptoms when deciding which intervention to use. The UP-A has been found to be efficacious in improving anxiety and depressive symptoms across open-trial, multiple-baseline, and RCT investigations (Ehrenreich et al., 2009; Ehrenreich-May et al., 2017; Trosper et al., 2009). The UP-A was initially tested using a multiple-baseline design. Three adolescents (aged 12 to 17 years) with principal anxiety or depressive disorders were included. These adolescents evidenced significant decreases in emotional disorder symptoms at post-treatment and continued improvement across six-month follow-up (Ehrenreich et al., 2009). These findings provided preliminary evidence of the UP-A in targeting emotional disorder symptoms (Ehrenreich et al., 2009). In an RCT with a waitlist comparison, 51 youth (aged 12 to 17 years) with a primary anxiety or depression diagnosis were randomized to receive the UP-A or waitlist control. Youth who completed UP-A evidenced lower diagnostic severity and greater global improvement compared to the waitlist condition at eight weeks and post-treatment (Ehrenreich-May et al., 2017). Child- and parent-rated outcomes also improved within this trial, but to a lesser degree than clinician-rated measures

(Ehrenreich-May et al., 2017). Ehrenreich-May et al. (2017) also assessed rates of change during and after treatment and found that those who participated in the UP-A showed significant improvement across outcome measures during and after treatment, although improvement after treatment was less rapid than during treatment. Similar to these findings, Queen et al. (2014) also found that youth included in both the open-trial and RCT investigations continued to show patterns of improvement in anxiety and depressive symptoms following treatment.

Prior studies have found the UP-C to be efficacious in improving anxiety and depressive symptoms in children aged seven to 12 years. The UP-C was originally created as a transdiagnostic group prevention program for anxiety and depression in youth (Ehrenreich-May & Bilek, 2011). This initial program investigated the utility of the Emotion Detectives Prevention Program (EDPP), a 15-session downward extension of and prevention framework for the UP, within a recreational summer camp setting. The prevention program included 40 youth (aged seven to 10 years) recruited from an existing recreational sports camp. Participants reported a significant decrease in anxiety symptoms post-prevention, with moderate to high participant satisfaction (Ehrenreich-May & Bilek, 2011). The EDPP was subsequently adapted into a group intervention for children with emotional disorders in order to specifically cater to clinical populations and maximize parental involvement, which had been relatively limited in the EDPP (Ehrenreich-May & Bilek, 2011). An initial open-trial investigation of the UP-C intervention included 22 youth (aged seven to 12 years) with principal anxiety diagnoses (with or without comorbid depressive symptoms/diagnoses), who completed 15 sessions of the UP-C. The researchers found significant improvements in clinician-rated anxiety and depression symptoms from pre- to post-treatment, with large effect sizes (Bilek & Ehrenreich-May, 2012). Kennedy et al. (2019) conducted a randomized controlled pilot trial of the UP-C with 47 children with a variety of emotional disorders, including anxiety, depression, and obsessive-compulsive-related disorders. These youth were randomly assigned to receive the UP-C or an established anxiety-focused group cognitive-behavioral intervention (Cool Kids; Lyneham et al., 2003). Youth were assessed prior to beginning treatment, eight weeks after starting treatment (mid-treatment), and 16 weeks after starting treatment (post-treatment). Youth in both conditions evidenced significant reductions in child- and parent-rated anxiety symptoms; however, youth in the UP-C condition demonstrated a more linear trajectory of improvement in parent-rated child depressive symptoms, as well as greater improvements in parent-rated youth sadness dysregulation and cognitive reappraisal from pre- to post-treatment (Kennedy et al., 2019). These findings suggested that the UP-C performed just as well as an established anxiety-specific group treatment in addressing anxiety symptoms and may also confer some additional benefits over anxiety-specific treatment in addressing depressive symptoms and emotion regulation. Adding to support for UP-C in addressing a range of emotional disorder diagnoses, Kennedy et al. (2018) found that the presence of a social anxiety disorder diagnosis was the only significant predictor of poorer UP-C treatment outcomes, consistent with a number of other cognitive-behavioral therapy protocols. This finding has led to potential modifications to the UP-C to target those with social anxiety earlier in the treatment, including greater exposure focus earlier in treatment, integration of social skills work, creating more opportunities for peer exposure, and a potentially longer course of treatment, among others.

Research has been conducted with the aim of attempting to capture different patterns of change across symptoms and across individuals as a result of the UP-C/A. Queen et al. (2014) found that youth- and parent-rated anxiety and depressive symptoms improved significantly during treatment, showing similar rates of improvement. Following treatment, youth-rated anxiety continued to show significant improvement, while depressive symptoms did not. Similarly, parent-rated anxiety and depressive symptoms did not change significantly following treatment (Queen et al., 2014). Kennedy et al. (2020) investigated trajectories of symptom changes following both the UP-C/A in a sample of 94 youth (aged seven to 17 years). Results provided support for the presence of three parent- and youth-reported response trajectories to the UP-C/A: an initial moderate severity class with steady improvement, an initial high severity class with rapid improvement, and an initial low severity class with steady improvement. Predictors of class status included pre-treatment symptom severity (e.g., less severe pre-treatment symptoms, better response), youth age (e.g., younger age, better response), and the presence of a social anxiety disorder diagnosis (e.g., better response if no social anxiety disorder). Sherman and Ehrenreich-May (2020) aimed to identify the timing in changes in potential risk/maintaining factors (e.g., distress tolerance, experiential avoidance, and cognitive flexibility) and link them to specific treatment components using eight adolescents with comorbid anxiety and depressive symptoms. Using single case analytics strategies, results suggested that parent-, child-, and clinician-rated symptoms improved significantly from pre- to post-treatment. Similarly, distress tolerance and avoidance also improved concurrently with symptom improvement (Sherman & Ehrenreich-May, 2020).

Currently, there are investigations under way or recently completed assessing the effectiveness of the UP-A in community mental health clinics in the United States and in Australia, as well as an ongoing waitlist-controlled RCT comparing the efficacy of the UP-A adapted as a universal, classroom-based preventive intervention in Spain to a waitlist control (García-Escalera et al., 2017; Jensen-Doss et al., 2018).

The UP-C and UP-A have been found to be efficacious for children and adolescents with a range of emotional concerns. In line with the criteria for evidence-based practices in psychology, they integrate best research evidence with clinical expertise and client values. They have been found to perform as well as established efficacious treatments for anxiety and depression concerns, with improvements shown compared to active and control conditions. They also demonstrate high feasibility and acceptability with youth, parents, and clinicians. The focus of the remaining chapters of this book will be the evidence for and application of these transdiagnostic treatments for specific client presentations.

REFERENCES

Barlow, D. H., Allen, L. B., & Choate, M. L. (2004). Toward a unified treatment for emotional disorders. *Behavior Therapy, 35*, 205–230.

Barlow, D. H., & Farchione, T. J. (Eds.). (2017). *Applications of the unified protocol for transdiagnostic treatment of emotional disorders.* Oxford University Press.

Barlow, D. H., Farchione, T. J., Bullis, J. R., Gallagher, M. W., Murray-Latin, H., Sauer-Zavala, S., Bentley, K. H., Thompson-Hollands, J., Conklin, L. R., Boswell, J. F., Ametaj, A., Carl, J. R., Boettcher, H. T, & Cassiello-Robbins, C. (2017a). The unified protocol for transdiagnostic treatment of emotional disorders compared with diagnosis-specific protocols for anxiety disorders: A randomized clinical trial. *JAMA Psychiatry, 74*(9), 875–884.

Barlow, D. H., Farchione, T. J., Sauer-Zavala, S., Latin, H. M., Ellard, K. K., Bullis, J. R. Bentley, K. H., Boettcher, H. T., & Cassiello-Robbins, C. (2017b). *Unified protocol for transdiagnostic treatment of emotional disorders: Therapist guide* (2nd ed). Oxford University Press.

Bentley, K. H., Sauer-Zavala, S., Cassiello-Robbins, C. F., Conklin, L. R., Vento, S., & Homer, D. (2017). Treating suicidal thoughts and behaviors within an emotional disorders framework: Acceptability and feasibility of the unified protocol in an inpatient setting. *Behavior Modification, 41*(4), 529–557.

Bilek, E. L., & Ehrenreich-May, J. (2012). An open trial investigation of a transdiagnostic group treatment for children with anxiety and depressive symptoms. *Behavior Therapy, 43*(4), 887–897. https://doi.org/10.1016/j.beth.2012.04.007

Chorpita, B. F., & Weisz, J. R. (2009). Modular Approach to Therapy for Children with Anxiety, Depression, Trauma, or Conduct problems (MATCH-ADTC). PracticeWise, LLC.

Chu, B. C. (2012). Translating transdiagnostic approaches to children and adolescents. *Cognitive and Behavioral Practice, 19*(1), 1–4. doi:https://doi.org/10.1016/j.cbpra.2011.06.003

Chu, B. C., Crocco, S. T., Esseling, P., Areizaga, M. J., Lindner, A. M., & Skriner, L. C. (2016). Transdiagnostic group behavioral activation and exposure therapy for youth anxiety and depression: Initial randomized controlled trial. *Behaviour Research and Therapy, 76*, 65–75.

Ehrenreich, J. T., Goldstein, C. M., Wright, L. R., & Barlow, D. H. (2009). Development of a unified protocol for the treatment of emotional disorders in youth. *Child & Family Behavior Therapy, 31*(1), 20–37. doi:10.1080/07317100802701228

Ehrenreich-May, J., & Bilek, E. L. (2011). Universal prevention of anxiety and depression in a recreational camp setting: An initial open trial. *Child and Youth Care Forum, 40*(6), 435–455. https://doi.org/10.1007/s10566-011-9148-4

Ehrenreich-May, J., Kennedy, S. M., Sherman, J. A., Bilek, E. L., Buzzella, B. A., Bennett, S. M., & Barlow, D. H. (2018). *Unified protocols for the transdiagnostic treatment of emotional disorders in children and adolescents: Therapist guide.* Oxford University Press.

Ehrenreich-May, J., Rosenfield, D., Queen, A. H., Kennedy, S. M., Remmes, C. S., & Barlow, D. H. (2017). An initial waitlist-controlled trial of the unified protocol for the treatment of emotional disorders in adolescents. *Journal of Anxiety Disorders, 46*, 46–55.

Ellard, K. K., Deckersbach, T., Sylvia, L. G., Nierenberg, A. A., & Barlow, D. H. (2012). Transdiagnostic treatment of bipolar disorder and comorbid anxiety with the unified protocol: A clinical replication series. *Behavior Modification, 36(4)*, 482–508.

Ellard, K. K., Fairholme, C. P., Boisseau, C. L., Farchione, T. J., & Barlow, D. H. (2010). Unified protocol for the transdiagnostic treatment of emotional disorders: Protocol development and initial outcome data. *Cognitive and Behavioral Practice, 17(1)*, 88–101. doi:http://dx.doi.org/10.1016/j.cbpra.2009.06.002

Fairburn, C. G., Cooper, Z., Doll, H. A., O'Connor, M. E., Bohn, K., Hawker, D. M., Wales, J. A., & Palmer, R. L. (2009). Transdiagnostic cognitive-behavioral therapy for patients with eating disorders: A two-site trial with 60-week follow-up. *American Journal of Psychiatry, 166(3)*, 311–319.

Fairburn, C. G., Cooper, Z., & Shafran, R. (2003). Cognitive behaviour therapy for eating disorders: A "transdiagnostic" theory and treatment. *Behaviour Research and Therapy, 41(5)*, 509–528.

Farchione, T. J., Fairholme, C. P., Ellard, K. K., Boisseau, C. L., Thompson-Hollands, J., Carl, J. R., Gallagher, M. W., & Barlow, D. H. (2012). Unified protocol for transdiagnostic treatment of emotional disorders: a randomized controlled trial. *Behavior Therapy, 43(3)*, 666–678. doi:10.1016/j.beth.2012.01.001

García-Escalera, J., Valiente, R. M., Chorot, P., Ehrenreich-May, J., Kennedy, S. M., & Sandín, B. (2017). The Spanish version of the unified protocol for transdiagnostic treatment of emotional disorders in adolescents (UP-A) adapted as a school-based anxiety and depression prevention program: Study protocol for a cluster randomized controlled trial. *JMIR Research Protocols, 6(8)*, e149–e149. doi:10.2196/resprot.7934

Harvey, A. G. (2016). A transdiagnostic intervention for youth sleep and circadian problems. *Cognitive and Behavioral Practice, 23(3)*, 341–355. doi:https://doi.org/10.1016/j.cbpra.2015.06.001

Jensen-Doss, A., Ehrenreich-May, J., Nanda, M. M., Maxwell, C. A., LoCurto, J., Shaw, A. M., Souer, H., Rosenfield, D., & Ginsburg, G. S. (2018). Community Study of Outcome Monitoring for Emotional Disorders in Teens (COMET): A comparative effectiveness trial of a transdiagnostic treatment and a measurement feedback system. *Contemporary Clinical Trials, 74*, 18–24. doi:https://doi.org/10.1016/j.cct.2018.09.011

Kennedy, S. M., Bilek, E. L., & Ehrenreich-May, J. (2019). A randomized controlled pilot trial of the unified protocol for transdiagnostic treatment of emotional disorders in children. *Behavior Modification, 43(3)*, 330–360.

Kennedy, S. M., Halliday, E. R., & Ehrenreich-May, J. (2020). Trajectories of Change and Intermediate Indicators of Non-Response to a Transdiagnostic Treatment for Children and Adolescents. *Journal of Clinical Child and Adolescent Psychology*, 1–15.

Kennedy, S. M., Tonarely, N. A., Sherman, J. A., & Ehrenreich-May, J. (2018). Predictors of treatment outcome for the unified protocol for transdiagnostic treatment of emotional disorders in children (UP-C). *Journal of Anxiety Disorders, 57*, 66–75.

Leichsenring, F., & Salzer, S. (2014). A unified protocol for the transdiagnostic psychodynamic treatment of anxiety disorders: An evidence-based approach. *Psychotherapy, 51(2)*, 224–245.

Loeb, K. L., Lock, J., Greif, R., & Le Grange, D. (2012). Transdiagnostic theory and application of family-based treatment for youth with eating disorders. *Cognitive and Behavioral Practice, 19(1)*, 17–30. doi:https://doi.org/10.1016/j.cbpra.2010.04.005

Lopez, M. E., Stoddard, J. A., Noorollah, A., Zerbi, G., Payne, L. A., Hitchcock, C. A., Meier, E., A., Esfahani, A. M., & Ray, D. B. (2015). Examining the efficacy of the unified protocol for transdiagnostic treatment of emotional disorders in the treatment of individuals with borderline personality disorder. *Cognitive and Behavioral Practice, 22*(4), 522–533.

Lyneham, H., Abbott, M., Wignall, A., & Rapee, R. (2003). *The Cool Kids anxiety treatment program.* Macquarie University.

Marchette, L. K., & Weisz, J. R. (2017). Practitioner review: Empirical evolution of youth psychotherapy toward transdiagnostic approaches. *Journal of Child Psychology and Psychiatry, 58(9)*, 970–984.

Newby, J. M., McKinnon, A., Kuyken, W., Gilbody, S., & Dalgleish, T. (2015). Systematic review and meta-analysis of transdiagnostic psychological treatments for anxiety and depressive disorders in adulthood. *Clinical Psychology Review, 40*, 91–110.

Norton, P. J., & Barrera, T. L. (2012). Transdiagnostic versus diagnosis-specific CBT for anxiety disorders: A preliminary randomized controlled noninferiority trial. *Depression and Anxiety, 29*(10), 874–882.

Norton, P. J., & Philipp, L. M. (2008). Transdiagnostic approaches to the treatment of anxiety disorders: A quantitative review. *Psychotherapy: Theory, Research, Practice, Training, 45*(2), 214.

Queen, A. H., Barlow, D. H., & Ehrenreich-May, J. (2014). The trajectories of adolescent anxiety and depressive symptoms over the course of a transdiagnostic treatment. *Journal of Anxiety Disorders, 28*(6), 511–521.

Sauer-Zavala, S., Bentley, K. H., & Wilner, J. G. (2016). Transdiagnostic treatment of borderline personality disorder and comorbid disorders: A clinical replication series. *Journal of Personality Disorders, 30*(1), 35–51.

Sauer-Zavala, S., Gutner, C. A., Farchione, T. J., Boettcher, H. T., Bullis, J. R., & Barlow, D. H. (2017). Current definitions of "transdiagnostic" in treatment development: A search for consensus. *Behavior Therapy, 48*(1), 128–138.

Sherman, J. A., & Ehrenreich-May, J. (2020). Changes in risk factors during the unified protocol for transdiagnostic treatment of emotional disorders in adolescents. *Behavior Therapy, 51*(6), 869–881.

Thompson-Brenner, H., Boswell, J. F., Espel-Huynh, H., Brooks, G., & Lowe, M. R. (2019). Implementation of transdiagnostic treatment for emotional disorders in residential eating disorder programs: A preliminary pre-post evaluation. *Psychotherapy Research, 29*(8), 1045–1061.

Trosper, S. E., Buzzella, B. A., Bennett, S. M., & Ehrenreich, J. T. (2009). Emotion regulation in youth with emotional disorders: Implications for a unified treatment approach. *Clinical Child and Family Psychology Review, 12*(3), 234–254.

PART 2

Applying the UP-C and UP-A to Specific Diagnoses and Problem Areas

4

Obsessive-Compulsive Disorder and Tic Disorder/ Tourette Syndrome

ASHLEY M. SHAW AND ELIZABETH R. HALLIDAY ■

OBSESSIVE-COMPULSIVE DISORDER

Overview

Obsessive-compulsive disorder (OCD) is characterized by obsessions and/ or compulsions that are frequent, distressing, and/or impairing (American Psychiatric Association [APA], 2013). Obsessions are typically followed by a compulsion, which is a repetitive behavior or mental act performed to reduce negative feelings (e.g., anxiety, guilt) associated with the obsession or to prevent a feared outcome (e.g., becoming ill or dying). This creates a negative reinforcement cycle, which maintains the frequency of obsessions and an exclusive reliance on compulsions for regulating emotions that arise from the obsession. Children and adolescents sometimes exhibit poor insight into their OCD symptoms (APA, 2013), which can provide a barrier to treatment engagement. Unfortunately, a striking 60% of childhood-onset cases persist into adulthood, making it essential to identify and effectively implement treatments for youth (APA, 2013). An estimated one-third to one-half of youth with OCD experience a comorbid anxiety disorder (Ivarsson et al., 2008; Langley et al., 2010). Additionally, 16% to 72% of youth with OCD experience lifetime major depressive disorder (MDD; Ortiz et al., 2016; Storch et al., 2012), and clients presenting with this comorbidity may be at elevated risk of treatment dropout (Aderka et al., 2011). Up to 30% of individuals with OCD have a lifetime tic disorder (TD; APA, 2013). The combination of comorbid OCD, TDs, and attention-deficit/hyperactivity disorder (ADHD) in children can pose unique treatment difficulties, such as aggression (APA, 2013; Debes et al., 2010). About half of youth with OCD also experience oppositional defiant disorder (ODD; Geller, 2006), and comorbid ADHD and ODD diagnoses are related to lower exposure and response prevention (ERP; the current gold standard for pediatric OCD) response rates (Storch et al., 2008). Researchers have also found that youth with comorbid OCD and MDD showed lower remission rates following traditional OCD treatment than those without MDD (Storch et al., 2008) and that trait anxiety also predicted worse treatment outcomes (Berman et al., 2000). Overall, comorbidities, such as MDD, ADHD, and ODD, can make engaging in OCD-specific treatment practices more challenging (Storch et al., 2008), which highlights the need for treatments that can target multiple comorbid disorders simultaneously.

Application of UP-C/A Case Conceptualization and Mechanisms to OCD

The UP-C/A posits that neuroticism underlies the co-occurrence among a range of emotional disorders (e.g., OCD, anxiety, and depression; Ehrenreich-May et al., 2018). Higher neuroticism has been implicated in OCD (e.g., Hofer et al., 2018). Relatedly, greater obsessive-compulsive symptoms (OCS) in youth have been linked to greater emotional lability and use of less adaptive emotion regulation skills, such as emotional suppression (Berman et al., 2018). Additionally, poor distress tolerance and a related construct, anxiety sensitivity (i.e., the fear of anxious sensations), may be unique mechanisms accounting for comorbidity between OCS and depression in youth (Chasson et al., 2017). Within the UP-C/A framework, compulsions are viewed as a maladaptive, rigidly applied emotion regulation strategy used to reduce uncomfortable feelings and are thus termed "emotional behaviors."

Adapting UP-C/A for OCD

The modular, flexible nature of the UP-C/A makes it feasible to apply to youth with OCD. Although many pediatric OCD treatments take as long as 20 sessions, we recently tested whether clients with OCD need more UP-C/A sessions than clients without OCD and found no significant differences between groups (Shaw et al., 2020). The average number of UP-C/A sessions for clients with OCD prior to discharge (n = 13) was almost 17 (Shaw et al., 2020), although symptom remission was not the only factor considered regarding termination and the termination decisions were not always a mutual decision between the therapist and the family (e.g., sometimes clients dropped out earlier than recommended). No major adaptations, such as modifications to handouts or incorporating other materials, are essential, although we will describe in what follows some material from

Franklin et al. (2018) that may be beneficial to use adjunctively. The UP-C/A may be most useful for youth with OCD who also experience co-occurring anxiety, depression, or anger/irritability. It may also be beneficial for OCD clients who perceive themselves as unable to tolerate an exclusive focus on ERP techniques or early exposure sessions or clients who have had a previous unsuccessful trial of ERP. Learning early UP-C/A skills prior to starting situational exposures may facilitate a more positive sense of treatment expectations and outcomes and help clients build self-efficacy to more aggressively address OCD symptoms with increasingly challenging exposures in the second half of treatment.

Table 4.1 provides an overview of UP-C/A content and suggested minor adaptations per module, whereas Table 4.2 compares how the content of the UP-C/A compares to a gold-standard cognitive-behavioral treatment for pediatric OCD with a heavy focus on ERP (Franklin et al., 2018). One major difference between the UP-C/A and this OCD-specific treatment is that the UP-C/A clinician does not need to provide diagnostic information or psychoeducation specifically about OCD to the child or adolescent. Rather, it is recommended to provide diagnostic feedback to the parent and use whatever language the child prefers to talk about their obsessions and compulsions. Coming up with their own wording to describe the OCD can be similar to "externalizing the OCD" (Franklin et al., 2018) for children, or it can be as simple as using their language (e.g., "scary thoughts") for adolescents. Avoiding the word and label of OCD in youth may be beneficial for youth who have poor insight, have low motivation for treatment, or are concerned about stigma.

In terms of module order, based on clinical experiences, we strongly recommend completing the "Emotional Behavior" form (typically completed in Module 7) earlier (e.g., during Module 3) to start working on opposite action as early as possible, and to facilitate checking in about opposite action practice throughout treatment. Although there are many different opposite actions that can be used in place of engaging in compulsions, the idea of "messing" with the rituals (e.g., delaying the ritual, setting a time limit on the ritual, doing the ritual out of order; Franklin et al., 2018) can be helpful for brainstorming opposite actions that proceed in the right direction toward eventual full response prevention. Module 3 is particularly important for clients with OCD who have depression or anger/irritability and may address some of the challenges that comorbidities (e.g., depression, ODD, ADHD) pose when treating pediatric OCD (Storch et al., 2008). Given that over one-third of children and 62% of adolescents with OCD experience depression (Geller, 2006), we believe the emotion-focused behavioral experiments for sadness (i.e., doing pleasant activities when down or bored) are important for youth with OCD, even when they are not currently in a major depressive episode.

Due to the flexibility of the UP-C/A, any later-module material can be moved earlier, particularly if it could be used as an opposite action for a compulsion (e.g., nonjudgmental awareness from Module 6). If clients are motivated, situational exposures can also be moved earlier. In terms of Module 5 (cognitive flexibility), it is important to normalize intrusive thoughts, by sharing the fact that from time to time everyone has unusual thoughts that they do not want or intend to act on.

Table 4.1 UP-C/A Adaptations for OCD and TDs

UP-A Module #	Recommended # of Sessions	UP-C/A Content	Adaptations for OCD and Tics
1	1–2	• Top Problems/goals • Explore motivation	• List Top Problems relevant to OCD and/or tics. • Figure out child's wording/language for their OCD.
2	1–2	• Emotion education • Breaking down emotions • Cycle of avoidance • "Tracking the Before, During, and After" form	• Increase recognition emotions that precede tics. • Compulsions = emotional behaviors • Discuss short- and long-term consequences of engaging in compulsions/tics.
3	2+	• Opposite action • Pleasant activity list • Emotion-focused behavior experiments	• Develop opposite actions to compulsions/tics, especially for those that are noticeable during session. • Ensure youth have activities they can engage in once compulsions are less time-consuming.
4	1	• Body drawing • Body scanning • Sensational exposures	• Identify and expose youth to physical sensations linked with intrusive thoughts, urges to ritualize, disgust. • Gain insight into sensations that accompany the premonitory urge.
5	2–3	• Thinking traps • Detective thinking • Problem solving	• Discuss thinking traps common to OCD (e.g., magical thinking) within UP-C/A and outside of it (e.g., thought–action fusion).
6	2	• Present-moment awareness • Nonjudgmental awareness • Generalized emotion exposures	• Use nonjudgmental awareness to let obsessions and premonitory urge pass without doing compulsion or tic. • Consider adding the "tic-specific sitting meditation."

Table 4.1 CONTINUED

UP-A Module #	Recommended # of Sessions	UP-C/A Content	Adaptations for OCD and Tics
7	2+	• "Emotional Behavior" form • Rationale for exposures • Situational exposures	• Do initial "Emotional Behavior" form in Module 3 to start opposite action practice early. • For OCD, conduct exposures with response prevention. • For tics, conduct exposures to antecedents of premonitory urge (e.g., stress, family conflict).
8	1–2	• Review • Relapse prevention	• For OCD, consider doing final sessions spaced two weeks to one month apart.
Parenting (P)	2+	• "Double Before, During, After" form • Emotional parenting behaviors: overprotection, criticism, inconsistency, modeling • Opposite parenting behaviors	• Utilize "Double Before, During, After" form to examine how family accommodation and parents' responses impact OCD and tics. • Reduce criticism, particularly if it triggers tics.

Although we have a comprehensive list of thinking traps in the UP-C/A, many of them relevant for OCD (e.g., magical thinking), during this module it may also be helpful to discuss thought–action fusion (i.e., the misconception that having a thought is equivalent to acting on the thought; Shafran & Rachman, 2004).

Recommended Usage of the UP-C/A for OCD

Preliminary research and our clinical experiences suggest that the UP-C and UP-A have multiple applications to OCD.

First, they can be used as a first-line intervention for youth with OCD who present with a variety of comorbid disorders, such as anxiety, depression, ODD, other obsessive-compulsive spectrum disorders (e.g., hoarding, excoriation disorder), and TDs. Our clinical experience suggests that using motivational interviewing and behavioral activation techniques early in the UP-C/A can overcome some of the obstacles to treating comorbid OCD and depression in youth.

Second, for youth with OCD alone who are unmotivated, have poor insight, or do not identify with the term OCD, the UP-C/A could be used as a first-line

Table 4.2 UP-C/A Content Compared to Traditional Cognitive-Behavioral Therapy (CBT) for Pediatric OCD

Treatment Component	UP-C/A	CBT for Pediatric OCD
Goal setting	✓	
Addressing motivation	✓Weighing My Options	✓"Story metaphors"
Psychoeducation	✓Regarding the function of emotions	✓Regarding OCD
Externalizing OCD		✓
Mapping OCD		✓
Feelings thermometer	✓Feelings thermometer	✓Fear thermometer
Functional analysis	✓"Tracking the Before, During, and After" form	✓Functional analysis focused on internal and external "triggers"
Opposite action	✓	✓"Breaking the rules of OCD"
Emotion-focused behavior experiments	✓	
Behavioral activation	✓Pleasant activity list	
Physical sensations	✓ Body drawing ✓ Body scanning ✓ Sensational exposures	✓
Thinking traps	✓	✓ Risk appraisal ✓ Over-responsibility
Cognitive restructuring	✓Detective thinking	✓ "Constructive self-talk" ✓ "Talking back to OCD"
Problem solving	✓	
Mindfulness	✓ Present-moment awareness ✓ Nonjudgmental awareness	✓"Detachment"
Generalized emotion exposures	✓	
Emotional behavior tracking	✓"Emotional Behavior" form	✓"Symptom list"
Exposures (situational and imaginal)		✓Exposure and response prevention
Relapse prevention	✓	✓
Functional analysis of parenting behaviors	✓"Double Before, During, After" form	
Parental behaviors	✓ Overprotection ✓ Criticism ✓ Inconsistency ✓ Modeling	✓ Criticism (i.e., "Stop giving advice") ✓ Accommodation of OCD ✓ Parental distress tolerance and anxiety
Opposite parenting behaviors, such as empathy, consistent rewards and punishment	✓	✓

Based on Franklin et al., 2018.

intervention (in a stepped-care approach) prior to moving into more intensive ERP work. Although such a sequenced approach has not yet been empirically examined, the first author frequently uses this approach in her clinical practice. For example, in treating a client with chronic OCD who insisted that he only experienced checking compulsions and mental rituals but not obsessions or any emotions attached to his OCD, the UP framework was utilized to first help him build awareness and acceptance of his emotions and thoughts prior to building a hierarchy and starting exposure work. Some ERP manuals (e.g., Franklin et al., 2018) emphasize labeling symptoms and behaviors as OCD, but the UP-C/A teaches youth to apply skills using general emotion language. This may be less aversive for certain youth who do not identify with the term OCD.

Third, the UP-C and UP-A may be particularly useful options for youth with OCD who have been non-responders to ERP, although no empirical studies have examined this. Given that the UP-C and UP-A focus on a wider variety of emotion regulation skills, youth with OCD may feel increased readiness for ERP after improving their distress tolerance with earlier modules of the UP-C/A.

Fourth, UP-C/A skills (e.g., emotion education, opposite action, problem solving, sensational exposures) can also be integrated into ERP. Including mindfulness practice into ERP treatment has been found to enhance treatment efficacy; thus, integrating present-moment and nonjudgmental awareness strategies into existing interventions might be particularly pertinent (Armstrong et al., 2013).

Empirical Support for the UP-C/A for OCD

Although there has been no randomized controlled trial (RCT) comparing the UP-C/A versus another intervention for OCD, studies applying the Unified Protocol for Transdiagnostic Treatment of Emotional Disorders (UP) to adults with primary OCD have demonstrated reduced OCD severity and equivalence between the UP and ERP in reducing OCD symptoms (e.g., Barlow et al., 2017a, 2017b). In a recent open trial investigating children and adolescents ($N = 170$; $n = 13$ had OCD) with an emotional disorder, youths' OCS decreased significantly, across child and parent report, regardless of child age or gender (Shaw et al., 2020). The researchers also found that youth with OCD did not differ from those without OCD on treatment engagement (e.g., premature dropout) or satisfaction (Shaw et al., 2020). While these results do not imply equivalence with existing ERP treatments, they provide preliminary support for the successful application of the UP-C/A to treat OCS in youth and suggest that the flexible structure of the UP-C/A may be useful for OCD.

Troubleshooting Barriers to Applying the UP-C/A to OCD

Applying the UP-C/A to OCD may be challenging for a therapist with less knowledge of OCD. For this reason, it may help to apply the UP-C/A to one case with anxiety or depression first to gain familiarity with the protocol prior to adapting it for OCD. Furthermore, we would recommend that any therapists with less knowledge of pediatric OCD educate themselves about OCD (see the psychoeducation resources aimed at parents in Franklin et al., 2018).

There may also be some challenges to using UP-C/A for clients with primary OCD in a group format. Specifically, some obsessions (e.g., about self-harm) may warrant doing exposures in private rather than in a shared space. Additionally, if the group comprises youth with a range of emotional disorder diagnoses, it is unlikely that in a mixed group, someone would have similar fears. To overcome this barrier, it is important to think ahead about the number of staff needed for groups. Specifically, for group sessions dedicated to exposure, we would recommend that clients with OCD have one-to-one therapist support.

Since the UP-A has one caregiver module (Module P) that can be flexibly used throughout treatment as needed, it is possible that caregivers of youth with OCD may need substantial parent-only work. Specifically, if parents have OCD themselves (e.g., contamination fears) that could intrude on the child's exposure homework (by either modeling fear or allowing avoidance), the therapist will likely have to spend more time providing rationale for specific exposures to parents and helping the parent model appropriate responses during exposures. Additionally, Module P will be needed if parents are struggling to reduce family accommodation of compulsions and other emotional behaviors.

Although we discussed some ways to personalize Module 5 for OCD (e.g., normalizing intrusive thoughts), cognitive reappraisal (termed detective thinking in the UP-C/A) can sometimes be challenging to apply to OCD, particularly if part of the client's ritual is researching/learning everything they need to know about their fears. Although some research has found that cognitive reappraisal is sometimes not the most useful technique for OCD (Tolin, 2009), detective thinking would be useful in addressing co-occurring depressive cognitions, fears of negative evaluation, and general worries. Indeed, there is evidence that utilizing cognitive strategies for non-OCD cognitions can enhance generalization and flexible thinking in relation to co-morbid anxiety disorders (March et al., 2007; Storch et al., 2008). Even if traditional cognitive restructuring does not go smoothly, our clinical experience and current gold-standard OCD treatments (Franklin et al., 2018) indicate that learning about and identifying thinking traps (e.g., magical thinking, thinking the worst) and/or developing a brief phrase to "boss back OCD" can still be particularly helpful. Thus, one streamlined session of Module 5, with a focus on thinking traps and "bossing back OCD," may be sufficient for clients with primary OCD, whereas Module 5 may take up to three sessions for clients with anxiety or depressive disorders.

AN OVERVIEW OF TIC DISORDERS

Clinicians have also begun to explore the potential utility of the UP-C/A for TDs. TDs and Tourette syndrome (TS), hereafter referred to inclusively as TDs, are neurological disorders that cause involuntary motor movements (e.g., blinking, shrugging shoulders) and/or sounds (e.g., humming, clearing throat, or yelling out a word or phrase; APA, 2013). Many people with TDs report premonitory urges, a sensation or urge to perform a motor or vocal activity; however, children identify this phenomenon less often than adults (Woods et al., 2005). The most common evidence-based psychosocial interventions for TS are behavior therapies (Himle & Capriotti, 2016; McGuire et al., 2014; Piacentini et al., 2010), such as habit reversal training (HRT) and the Comprehensive Behavioral Intervention for Tics (CBIT; Leckman et al., 1991; Whittington et al., 2016). The initial goal of behavioral therapies for TDs is to identify the antecedents, or "tic triggers," and consequences that worsen tics. The main goals of behavioral strategies for TDs are to eliminate, reduce, or change the antecedents and consequences of tics to most effectively decrease the intensity, frequency, complexity, and situational fluctuation of interfering tics.

Application of UP-C/A Case Conceptualization and Mechanisms to TDs

Youth with TDs experience high rates of comorbidities, including OCD, anxiety disorders, ODD, ADHD, and depression (Bloch et al., 2009). Unfortunately, comorbidities are often overlooked in TDs because observable tics can overshadow the severity and impairment of other disorders (Coffey et al., 2000). Studies have demonstrated that comorbidity often causes more problems than the tics themselves (Pile et al., 2018; Storch et al., 2007). Given these comorbidity patterns, it is unsurprising that youth with TDs have been found to have higher levels of neuroticism and related avoidant coping styles (i.e., social withdrawal) compared to those without TDs (Chen et al., 2005; Wang et al., 2008). Many youth with TDs also struggle with anger (Budman et al., 2000; Lebowitz et al., 2012). Tics are also worsened by experiences of heightened negative and positive emotions, including exhaustion, anxiety, stress, and excitement (e.g., taking a test, participating in exciting activities; Capriotti et al., 2015). The UP-C/A can help youth with TDs learn to modify how various antecedents (e.g., strong emotions) impact their responses, with the goal to teach youth how to allow the emotion or premonitory urge to exist without engaging in the tic.

Adapting the UP-C/A for TDs

In terms of adapting the UP-C/A for TDs, some of the recommended adaptations are outlined in Box 4.1. In our work thus far with clients with TDs, we have not adapted any of the handouts. In Module 2, starting to monitor and attend to tics during session will help the therapist and client identify potential triggers for tics, and later practice incorporating an opposite action. It may be helpful for therapists to discuss not-just-right feelings during emotion education, particularly if the child's tics are not always linked to more common strong emotions (e.g., anxiety, anger, excitement) or stress. Additionally, the "Tracking the Before, During, and After" form should be completed repeatedly until all antecedents (i.e., the "Before") and consequences (i.e., the "After") of the tic have been identified. In Module 3, the term "opposite action" can be used akin to the term "competing response" in HRT and CBIT. One of the major modifications to traditional UP-C/A would be that opposite action practice for tics should be reviewed, attended to during session (when tics arise), and assigned for homework every week. If the client is not currently depressed, behavioral experiments for sadness and pleasant activity scheduling might be more helpful to boost self-esteem, given that tics can negatively impact self-esteem. In Module 4, the therapist should help the client identify what sensations arise during a premonitory urge. For example, they might use the body drawing to draw where they feel the premonitory urge. The therapist should also encourage using body scanning during a premonitory urge to identify which sensations are occurring that lead to engaging in the tic. Sensations that arise during a premonitory urge could also be elicited with sensational exposures.

Based on recent preliminary research supporting using mindfulness-based stress reduction for teens and adults with TDs (Reese et al., 2015), Module 6 content might be particularly beneficial for youth with TDs. Given this research, it would be helpful to add a "tic-specific sitting meditation," which allows clients to practice mindfully noticing urges to tic, riding the urge "like a wave," and "anchoring oneself to the breath" without engaging in the tic or trying to change the urge (Reese et al., 2015). For Module 7, if stress increases tics for the child, exposures should be used to practice acting opposite of the tic even in the face of various stressors (e.g., receiving negative feedback, discussing a difficult topic with their parent, taking a test; Conelea et al., 2011).

In terms of Module P, clinicians often find that parents' own emotions or inability to tolerate the distress and social stigma of their child's tics contribute to antecedents and consequences that further maintain their child's tics. Empathy, understanding, and "tic-neutral" environments (e.g., reducing reinforcement for tics at home, including limiting excessive attention to the tics and using discreet signals to prompt competing responses rather than parents becoming "tic police") often need to be emphasized to maintain a positive approach to treatment of tics in youth (Conelea & Woods, 2008; Franklin et al., 2012). It seems important to explore parents' emotional behaviors as potential triggers for tics and how parents' responses to tics impact tic recurrence. Parents should be taught the "Double Before, During, After" form to explore their responses to their child's tics, and whether it makes sense for them to prompt an opposite action or engage in planned ignoring.

Empirical Support and Recommended Usage of UP-C/A for TDs

Research is needed on the efficacy of the UP-C/A for TDs and which treatment components are most useful, for whom, and in which combination or order. In a published open-trial investigation of the UP-C, two youths (12.5% of sample) had comorbid TDs (Bilek & Ehrenreich-May, 2012). In a more recent study of the UP-C/A, three participants had a primary TD (3.2% of the sample) and two participants (2.1% of the sample) had comorbid TDs and demonstrated improved outcomes for co-occurring internalizing symptoms (Kennedy et al., 2020). The UP-C/A may be most appropriately used when TDs are a secondary rather than a primary diagnosis or as an adjunctive or alternative intervention for CBIT non-responders. UP-C/A treatment strategies could also be incorporated into CBIT/HRT. Overall, the presence and severity of comorbid diagnoses should be considered when deciding if the UP-C/A should be considered and when (e.g., before or after CBIT). To summarize how the UP-C/A can be applied to OCD and TDs, refer to the tip sheets later in the chapter.

CASE EXAMPLE OF USING THE UP-A FOR A CHILD WITH OCD AND TS

Here we outline the case of Carlos, a 12-year-old, White, Hispanic/Latinx male who was treated with the UP-A. With his mother Carlos completed a pre-treatment intake that included a semistructured diagnostic interview, the Anxiety Disorders Interview Schedule for DSM-5 Child and Parent versions (ADIS-5 C/P; Silverman & Albano, 1996, in press). He received a principal diagnosis of OCD and additional diagnoses of TS, generalized anxiety disorder (GAD), and social anxiety disorder. Carlos was not taking any medication at the intake or during treatment. Carlos's OCD included unacceptable thoughts (e.g., about hurting himself and others), rewriting/re-reading, and checking. Specifically, Carlos reported having intrusive thoughts and images about hurting his family, friends, or himself multiple times a day (e.g., shooting himself and his family). Carlos reported that he tried to neutralize these thoughts by thinking of his "happy place," as well as staying close to and calling his family members. Carlos also reported writing and rewriting assignments because they do not look correct, checking his grades excessively, and repeatedly checking his answers on tests. Due to his intrusive thoughts, Carlos reported spending less time with peers and having difficulty concentrating at school. Carlos's TS diagnosis was assigned to account for his persistent vocal tics (i.e., sniffing, snorting, coughing, and blurting out syllables and song lyrics) and motor tics (i.e., "cracking" his neck, toes, and elbow).

Carlos completed 21 sessions of individual UP-A. Notably, Carlos's parents did not accommodate his OCD, did not serve as a trigger or reinforcer of his tics, and did not have many emotional parenting behaviors. Due to this as well as Carlos's good insight and strong motivation, most session work was done with him, with parent check-ins during five to 10 minutes of each session. During initial sessions, the therapist and Carlos developed Top Problems (Module 1), which included working on his "scary thoughts." During goal setting, the therapist discussed how, rather than setting a goal to "get rid of scary thoughts," they would develop more adaptive ways for him to manage the thoughts. Carlos practiced emotion identification and learned to break down his emotional response following the trigger of "scary thoughts" (i.e., the "Tracking the Before, During, and After" form; Module 2). Following "scary thoughts," he shared that he felt sad and scared, distracted himself, and thought about his "happy place" (i.e., "During" the emotional response). Also, the therapist briefly introduced detective thinking (typically covered in Module 5) by discussing what the cycle of thoughts, feelings, and behaviors would look like if he thought "Oh, that's silly, I would never do that" instead of "These thoughts are bad because I know I shouldn't do it." The therapist also provided psychoeducation to his mother about OCD (Franklin et al., 2018).

Sessions 3 through 5 focused on using detective thinking (Module 5) and present-moment awareness (Module 6) to act opposite (Module 3). For example, the therapist supported Carlos in reframing negative interpretations of his intrusive thoughts. They also completed an "Emotional Behavior" form (usually completed in Module 7) early on to start working on opposite actions for compulsions and tics. Some emotional behaviors included avoiding "dangerous places," crowded malls, violent TV and video games, and being alone when he has intrusive thoughts. They planned opposite actions, including telling himself "I'm OK with these thoughts" and practicing present-moment awareness (i.e., noticing three things around him to anchor himself to the present moment). Present-moment awareness was introduced early to facilitate its use as an opposite action. For his neck twitch, his opposite action was to "straighten his posture."

Remaining sessions focused on Modules 5 and 7. For example, the therapist and Carlos practiced identifying thinking traps, detective thinking, and problem solving. They frequently updated his "Emotional Behavior" form. The therapist presented the rationale for exposure and created an emotion ladder around checking and question-asking behaviors related to his schoolwork. Then they completed a test-taking exposure in which he could only check his work once, could not ask how he did, and could not check the internet later for the meaning of a word. The therapist also conducted an exposure around writing an essay without being able to rewrite it or correct himself. By Session 18, the therapist considered making an emotion ladder for lingering OCD concerns, but Carlos denied that any triggers related to his OCD still provoked strong emotions and that any of the associated emotional behaviors were still frequent. Approximately five sessions focused on exposures for social anxiety and GAD. At termination (Module 8), Carlos and his mother reported improvements across Top Problems and symptoms. They reported that his "scary thoughts" had decreased significantly and that his main motor tic (a neck twitch) had also been reduced. Diagnostic impressions were that OCD had fully remitted and subthreshold symptoms of GAD, social anxiety, and TS remained. Overall, Carlos and his mother were very satisfied with treatment. Carlos reported that opposite action and detective thinking were the most helpful skills he learned.

SUMMARY

This chapter outlined the clinical utility of the UP-C/A for treating youth with OCD and TDs, particularly when comorbid anxiety or depression is present. Some suggested adaptations include starting opposite action practice as early as possible and assigning it for homework throughout modules and potentially incorporating psychoeducation from Franklin et al. (2018) for both children and parents. In terms of order, we recommend that the UP-C/A be applied in a flexible order for OCD, such as doing the "Emotional Behavior" form early on, introducing non-judgmental awareness as early as seems relevant, and doing exposures as soon as the client is ready.

Tip Sheet for Using UP-C and UP-A in Youth with OCD

✓ **Why use UP-C and UP-A for OCD?**
  - The UP-C/A can simultaneously address common comorbid diagnoses and intense emotions (e.g., depression, anger, and irritability) that may make using straightforward exposure and response prevention more challenging.
  - Preliminary research has suggested that youth with OCD exhibit transdiagnostic emotional vulnerabilities (e.g., emotional lability and less adaptive emotion regulation skills) that can be targeted in the UP-C/A.
  - The UP-C/A can be helpful for youth with OCD who are initially unmotivated, are hesitant to engage in exposure, have poor insight, and/or are concerned about stigma. The UP-C/A addresses these barriers by utilizing motivational interviewing strategies, avoiding diagnostic labels, and teaching youth a variety of emotion regulation skills to increase distress tolerance before starting exposure.
  - The UP-C/A incorporate mindfulness techniques, such as nonjudgmental and present-moment awareness, which can be helpful responses to obsessions and opposite actions in place of engaging in compulsions.

✓ **How do I use UP-C and UP-A for OCD?**
  - Break down the emotional experience of obsessions and compulsions by labeling intrusive thoughts as "triggers," obsessions as "thoughts," and compulsions as "emotional behaviors" (Module 2).
  - Complete the "Emotional Behavior" form (typically completed in Module 7) earlier (e.g., during Module 3) to start working on opposite action as early as possible and to facilitate checking in about opposite action practice throughout treatment.
  - Conduct behavioral experiments to test whether the child can effectively implement opposite actions (e.g., assist the child in completing a behavioral experiment to see what happens if, instead of washing their hands right after they touch the door, they wait 15 minutes; Module 3).
  - Use nonjudgmental awareness to let obsessions pass without doing the compulsion.
  - If appropriate, begin Module 7 early to provide more exposure practice.
  - Home learning practice is especially important for OCD. Skills should be practiced frequently and consistently in multiple different settings.

✓ **What challenges might come up when using UP-C and UP-A for OCD?**
  - Children and adolescents may not feel motivated to address their behaviors or may not understand or be able to articulate their obsessions.

✓ **When is UP-C or UP-A not appropriate for youth with OCD?**

- If a child or teen is *only* experiencing OCD symptoms, with no other comorbidities, and is motivated to engage in exposure therapy, a single-disorder approach (e.g., Franklin et al., 2018) may be more appropriate.
- Additionally, although the UP-C/A has been used clinically with youth with mild to moderate OCD, it has not yet been applied to youth with severe OCD.

Tip Sheet for Using UP-C and UP-A in Youth with TDs

✓ **Why use UP-C and UP-A for TDs?**
- The UP-C/A can address comorbid disorders and intense emotions common in youth with TDs (e.g., depression, anxiety, anger). Both intense negative and positive emotions can exacerbate tics.
- Youth with TDs also exhibit some emotional vulnerabilities (e.g., social withdrawal, sensory intolerances) that can be targeted with the UP-C/A.
- The UP-C/A can help youth with TDs learn to modify how various antecedents (e.g., strong emotions) impact their responses, with the goal to teach youth to allow the emotions or premonitory urge to exist without engaging in the tic.

✓ **How do I use UP-C and UP-A for TDs?**
- Emotion education in Module 2 can be applied to tics as follows:
  - The trigger is anything that precedes the tic (e.g., sitting in class, taking a test, watching TV, reading).
  - Body clues/sensations are the premonitory urge to perform the tic.
  - The emotional behavior is the tic.
- Use the "Tracking the Before, During, and After" (BDA) form (Module 2) and the "Double BDA" form (Module P) to help the youth and their caregiver develop insight into situations or emotions that increase tics and short- and long-term consequences that reinforce tics. The BDA should be completed repeatedly until all antecedents (i.e., the "Before") and consequences (i.e., the "After") of the tic have been identified.
- Introduce opposite action to performing tics (also known as "competing response") in response to the urge as early as possible (e.g., in Module 3).
- If a premonitory urge is present, use sensational exposures and/or present-moment awareness to increase tolerance to the urge (Module 4).
- Problem-solving is helpful to address interpersonal difficulties that contribute to anxiety, anger, or fatigue, which may increase tics (Module 5).
- Situational exposure practice should focus on other emotional problems experienced by the child or exposing the child to the antecedents of tics while having them practice their opposite action (Module 7).
- Use opposite parenting behaviors for caregivers who exhibit overprotection/overcontrol (e.g., excusing child from dinner table due to tics; Module P).

✓ **What challenges might come up when using UP-C and UP-A for TDs?**
- When utilizing caregivers to prompt the child's opposite action, you may need to facilitate a discussion about the most helpful way to do this and how a caregiver can use empathy in this role.

- Since children are less likely to identify a premonitory urge than adults, it may be challenging to identify body clues.

✓ **When is UP-C or UP-A not appropriate for youth with TDs?**

- Individuals participating in treatment with TDs are appropriate candidates for the UP-C/A if they also have an emotional disorder. Emotion education materials are geared toward these symptoms rather than tics.
- For youth who do not present with any emotional disorder comorbidities, a targeted treatment (e.g., habit reversal, Comprehensive Behavioral Intervention for Tics [CBIT]) is more appropriate.

REFERENCES

Aderka, I. M., Anholt, G. E., van Balkom, A. J., Smit, J. H., Hermesh, H., Hofmann, S. G., & van Oppen, P. (2011). Differences between early and late drop-outs from treatment for obsessive-compulsive disorder. *Journal of Anxiety Disorders, 25*(7), 918–923. doi:10.1016/j.janxdis.2011.05.004

American Psychiatric Association. (2013). *Diagnostic and statistical manual of mental disorders* (5th ed.). American Psychiatric Publishing.

Armstrong, A. B., Morrison, K. L., & Twohig, M. P. (2013). A preliminary investigation of acceptance and commitment therapy for adolescent obsessive-compulsive disorder. *Journal of Cognitive Psychotherapy, 27*(2), 175–190.

Barlow, D. H., Farchione, T. J., Bullis, J. R., Gallagher, M. W., Murray-Latin, H., Sauer-Zavala, S., Bentley, K. H., Thompson-Hollands, J., Conklin, L. R., Boswell, J. F., Ametaj, A., Carl, J. R., Boettcher, H. T, & Cassiello-Robbins, C. (2017a). The unified protocol for transdiagnostic treatment of emotional disorders compared with diagnosis-specific protocols for anxiety disorders: A randomized clinical trial. *JAMA Psychiatry, 74*(9), 875–884.

Barlow, D. H., Farchione, T. J., Sauer-Zavala, S., Latin, H. M., Ellard, K. K., Bullis, J. R., Bentley, K.H., Boettcher, H.T., & Cassiello-Robbins, C. (2017b). *Unified protocol for transdiagnostic treatment of emotional disorders: Therapist guide:* Oxford University Press.

Berman, N. C., Shaw, A. M., Curley, E. E., & Wilhelm, S. (2018). Emotion regulation and obsessive-compulsive phenomena in youth. *Journal of Obsessive-Compulsive and Related Disorders, 19*, 44–49. doi:10.1016/j.jocrd.2018.07.005

Berman, S. L., Weems, C. F., Silverman, W. K., & Kurtines, W. M. (2000). Predictors of outcome in exposure-based cognitive and behavioral treatments for phobic and anxiety disorders in children. *Behavior Therapy, 31*(4), 713–731.

Bilek, E. L., & Ehrenreich-May, J. (2012). An open trial investigation of a transdiagnostic group treatment for children with anxiety and depressive symptoms. *Behavior Therapy, 43*(4), 887–897.

Bloch, M. H., & Leckman, J. F. (2009). Clinical course of Tourette syndrome. *Journal of Psychosomatic Research, 67*(6), 497–501.

Budman, C. L., Bruun, R. D., Park, K. S., Lesser, M., & Olson, M. (2000). Explosive outbursts in children with Tourette's disorder. *Journal of the American Academy of Child & Adolescent Psychiatry, 39*(10), 1270–1276.

Capriotti, M. R., Piacentini, J. C., Himle, M. B., Ricketts, E. J., Espil, F. M., Lee, H. J., Turkel, J. E., & Woods, D. W. (2015). Assessing environmental consequences of ticcing in youth with chronic tic disorders: The Tic Accommodation and Reactions Scale. *Children's Health Care, 44*(3), 205–220.

Chasson, G. S., Bello, M. S., Luxon, A. M., Graham, T. A., & Leventhal, A. M. (2017). Transdiagnostic emotional vulnerabilities linking obsessive-compulsive and depressive symptoms in a community-based sample of adolescents. *Depression and Anxiety, 34*(8), 761–769.

Chen, Y., Chunyan, W., Lifang, M., Jiang, D., Jing, L., & Wang, X. (2005). Behavior disorders and personality in children with tic disorders. *Chinese Journal of Clinical Rehabilitation, 9*(20), 232–234.

Coffey, B. J., Biederman, J., Geller, D. A., Spencer, T. J., Kim, G. S., Bellordre, C. A., Frazier, J. A., Cradock, K., & Magovcevic, M. (2000). Distinguishing illness severity from tic severity in children and adolescents with Tourette's disorder. *Journal of the American Academy of Child & Adolescent Psychiatry, 39*(5), 556–561.

Conelea, C. A., & Woods, D. W. (2008). The influence of contextual factors on tic expression in Tourette's syndrome: A review. *Journal of Psychosomatic Research, 65*(5), 487–496.

Conelea, C. A., Woods, D. W., & Brandt, B. C. (2011). The impact of a stress induction task on tic frequencies in youth with Tourette Syndrome. *Behaviour Research and Therapy, 49*(8), 492–497.

Debes, N., Hjalgrim, H., & Skov, L. (2010). The presence of attention-deficit hyperactivity disorder (ADHD) and obsessive-compulsive disorder worsen psychosocial and educational problems in Tourette syndrome. *Journal of Child Neurology, 25*(2), 171–181.

Ehrenreich-May, J., Bilek, E., Buzzella, B., Kennedy, S., Mash, J., Bennett, S., & Barlow, D. (2018). *Unified protocols for the treatment of emotional disorders in adolescents (UP-A) and children (UP-C): Therapist guide.* Oxford University Press.

Franklin, M. E., Freeman, J. B., & March, J. S. (2018). *Treating OCD in children and adolescents: A cognitive-behavioral approach.* Guilford.

Franklin, M. E., Harrison, J. P., & Benavides, K. L. (2012). Obsessive-compulsive and tic-related disorders. *Child and Adolescent Psychiatric Clinics, 21*(3), 555–571.

Geller, D. A. (2006). Obsessive-compulsive and spectrum disorders in children and adolescents. *Psychiatric Clinics of North America, 29*(2), 353–370. doi:10.1016/j.psc.2006.02.012

Himle, M. B., & Capriotti, M. R. (2016). Behavioral therapy for Tourette disorder: An update. *Current Behavioral Neuroscience Reports, 3*(3), 211–217.

Hofer, P. D., Wahl, K., Meyer, A. H., Miché, M., Beesdo-Baum, K., Wittchen, H.-U., & Lieb, R. (2018). The role of behavioral inhibition, perceived parental rearing, and adverse life events in adolescents and young adults with incident obsessive-compulsive disorder. *Journal of Obsessive-Compulsive and Related Disorders, 19*, 116–123.

Ivarsson, T., Melin, K., & Wallin, L. (2008). Categorical and dimensional aspects of comorbidity in obsessive-compulsive disorder (OCD). *European Child & Adolescent Psychiatry, 17*(1), 20–31. doi:10.1007/s00787-007-0626-z

Kennedy, S. M., Halliday, E., & Ehrenreich-May, J. (2020). Trajectories of change and intermediate indicators of non-response to transdiagnostic treatment for children and adolescents. *Journal of Clinical Child & Adolescent Psychology*, 1–15 [online before print]. doi:10.1080/15374416.2020.1716363

Langley, A. K., Lewin, A. B., Bergman, R. L., Lee, J. C., & Piacentini, J. (2010). Correlates of comorbid anxiety and externalizing disorders in childhood obsessive compulsive disorder. *European Child & Adolescent Psychiatry, 19*(8), 637–645.

Lebowitz, E. R., Motlagh, M. G., Katsovich, L., King, R. A., Lombroso, P. J., Grantz, H., Lin, H., Bentley, M. J., Gilbert, D. L., Singer, H. S., Coffey, B. J. Tourette Syndrome Study Group, Kurlan, R. M., & Leckman, J. F. (2012). Tourette syndrome in youth with and without obsessive compulsive disorder and attention deficit hyperactivity disorder. *European Child & Adolescent Psychiatry, 21*(8), 451–457.

Leckman, J. F., Hardin, M. T., Riddle, M. A., Stevenson, J., Ort, S. I., & Cohen, D. (1991). Clonidine treatment of Gilles de la Tourette's syndrome. *Archives of General Psychiatry, 48*(4), 324–328.

March, J. S., Franklin, M. E., Leonard, H., Garcia, A., Moore, P., Freeman, J., & Foa, E. (2007). Tics moderate treatment outcome with sertraline but not cognitive-behavior therapy in pediatric obsessive-compulsive disorder. *Biological Psychiatry, 61*(3), 344–347.

McGuire, J. F., Piacentini, J., Brennan, E. A., Lewin, A. B., Murphy, T. K., Small, B. J., & Storch, E. A. (2014). A meta-analysis of behavior therapy for Tourette syndrome. *Journal of Psychiatric Research, 50*, 106–112.

Ortiz, A., Morer, A., Moreno, E., Plana, M., Cordovilla, C., & Lázaro, L. (2016). Clinical significance of psychiatric comorbidity in children and adolescents with obsessive-compulsive disorder: Subtyping a complex disorder. *European Archives of Psychiatry & Clinical Neuroscience, 266*(3), 199–208.

Piacentini, J., Woods, D. W., Scahill, L., Wilhelm, S., Peterson, A. L., Chang, S., Ginsburg, G. S., Deckersbach, T., Dziura, J., Levi-Pearl, S., & Walkup, J. T. (2010). Behavior therapy for children with Tourette disorder: A randomized controlled trial. *Journal of the American Medical Association, 303*(19), 1929–1937.

Pile, V., Lau, J. Y., Topor, M., Hedderly, T., & Robinson, S. (2018). Interoceptive accuracy in youth with tic disorders: Exploring links with premonitory urge, anxiety and quality of life. *Journal of Autism and Developmental Disorders, 48*(10), 3474–3482.

Reese, H. E., Vallejo, Z., Rasmussen, J., Crowe, K., Rosenfield, E., & Wilhelm, S. (2015). Mindfulness-based stress reduction for Tourette syndrome and chronic tic disorder: A pilot study. *Journal of Psychosomatic Research, 78*(3), 293–298. doi:10.1016/j.jpsychores.2014.08.001

Shafran, R., & Rachman, S. (2004). Thought-action fusion: A review. *Journal of Behavior Therapy and Experimental Psychiatry, 35*(2), 87–107. doi:10.1016/j.jbtep.2004.04.002

Shaw, A. M., Halliday, E. R., & Ehrenreich-May, J. (2020). The effect of transdiagnostic emotion-focused treatment on obsessive-compulsive symptoms in children and adolescents. *Journal of Obsessive-Compulsive and Related Disorders, 26*, 100552.

Silverman, W. K., & Albano, A. M. (1996). *Anxiety Disorders Interview Schedule for DSM-IV, Child & Parent Versions*. Psychological Corporation.

Silverman, W. K., & Albano, A. M. (in press). *Anxiety Disorders Interview Schedule for DSM-5, Child & Parent Versions*.

Storch, E. A., Lewin, A. B., Larson, M. J., Geffken, G. R., Murphy, T. K., & Geller, D. (2012). Depression in youth with obsessive-compulsive disorder: Clinical phenomenology and correlates. *Psychiatry Research, 196*(1), 83–89.

Storch, E. A., Merlo, L. J., Lack, C., Milsom, V. A., Geffken, G. R., Goodman, W. K., & Murphy, T. K. (2007). Quality of life in youth with Tourette's syndrome and chronic tic disorder. *Journal of Clinical Child & Adolescent Psychiatry, 36*(2), 217–227.

Storch, E. A., Merlo, L. J., Larson, M. J., Geffken, G. R., Lehmkuhl, H. D., Jacob, M. L., Murphy, T. K., & Goodman, W. K. (2008). Impact of comorbidity on cognitive-behavioral therapy response in pediatric obsessive-compulsive disorder. *Journal of the American Academy of Child & Adolescent Psychiatry, 47*(5), 583–592.

Tolin, D. F. (2009). Alphabet soup: ERP, CT, and ACT for OCD. *Cognitive and Behavioral Practice, 16*(1), 40–48.

Wang, P., Wang, X.-W., Huang, C.-L., & Yang, X.-W. (2008). Analysis of personality characteristics of children with Tourette's syndrome. *Chinese Journal of Child Health Care, 4*, 447–449.

Whittington, C., Pennant, M., Kendall, T., Glazebrook, C., Trayner, P., Groom, M., Hedderly, T., Heyman, I., Jackson, G., Jackson, S. Murphy, T., Rickards, H.,

Robertson, M., Stern, J., & Hollis, C. (2016). Practitioner review: Treatments for Tourette syndrome in children and young people—a systematic review. *Journal of Child Psychology and Psychiatry, 57*(9), 988–1004.

Woods, D. W., Piacentini, J., Himle, M. B., & Chang, S. (2005). Premonitory Urge for Tics Scale (PUTS): Initial psychometric results and examination of the premonitory urge phenomenon in youths with tic disorders. *Journal of Developmental & Behavioral Pediatrics, 26*(6), 397–403.

5

Pediatric Irritability and Disruptive Behaviors

JESSICA LYN HAWKS, SARAH M. KENNEDY, AND JACOB BENJAMIN WESTRICK HOLZMAN ■

PEDIATRIC IRRITABILITY

Irritability is defined as having a low threshold for experiencing anger in response to frustration and has two components: tonic and phasic. The tonic component refers to being persistently angry/grumpy, while the phasic component refers to behavioral outbursts of intense anger (Moore et al., 2019). Pediatric irritability is considered a transdiagnostic symptom dimension that exists across several psychiatric disorders diagnosed in youth (Evans et al., 2017). Persistent irritability is a diagnostic criterion for several externalizing disorders within the fifth edition of the *Diagnostic and Statistical Manual of Mental Disorders* (DSM-5), including intermittent explosive disorder and oppositional defiant disorder, as well as internalizing disorders, including disruptive mood dysregulation disorder, major depressive disorder, and generalized anxiety disorder (American Psychiatric Association, 2013).

Approximately 3.3% of community youth experience significant rates of irritability (Brotman et al., 2017). Additionally, irritability and its related constructs (e.g., anger, frustration, aggression) are the most common reason youth are referred for mental health services (Brotman et al., 2006). Importantly, after the preschool period, levels of irritability tend to remain relatively stable and are predictive of anxiety and depressive disorders into adulthood. In fact, research has shown the presence of significant irritability in childhood is more predictive of depression in adulthood than is the presence of a depressive disorder in childhood (Brotman et al., 2006). Given the relatively high prevalence of irritability in childhood and the strong presence of irritability across a spectrum of psychiatric disorders, it is imperative to develop clinical interventions that can address irritability from a transdiagnostic perspective to improve outcomes while working with this client population.

CONCEPTUALIZING IRRITABILITY AND DISRUPTIVE BEHAVIORS FROM A TRANSDIAGNOSTIC PERSPECTIVE

Transdiagnostic models consider underlying mechanisms as transdiagnostic when such factors influence the development and/or maintenance of multiple presenting concerns (Ehrenreich-May & Chu, 2014). Such underlying mechanisms may exist at both individual (i.e., child-focused) and contextual (i.e., parent- and environment-focused) levels (Nolen-Hoeksema & Watkins, 2011). Several transdiagnostic mechanisms are implicated in the development and maintenance of irritability and associated disruptive behaviors in youth, including information processing biases (Reid et al., 2006), dispositions for high negative emotional reactivity (Eisenberg et al., 2001), use of escape-based strategies in response to negative emotions (Patterson, 1982), and parenting practices (Kolko et al., 2008).

A transactional model of child development (Patterson, 1982) highlights how both child-focused and contextual factors are implicated in the development and maintenance of irritability and disruptive behaviors. Patterson's (1982) co-ercive family processes model highlights how parent–child interactions that reinforce emotional lability and avoidance-based coping strategies are involved in the development and course of irritability and disruptive behaviors in youth. For example, a parent may make repeated requests of a noncompliant child, while often modeling significant irritability (e.g., yelling). Eventually, as the parent's negative affective state worsens, they withdraw their request in response to their child's irritability and noncompliant behaviors. In doing so, the parent negatively reinforces their child's noncompliance and irritability by withdrawing the aversive command. The parent's avoidant behavior (i.e., withdrawing command) is also negatively reinforced by the cessation of the child's irritability and disruptive behaviors. This cycle is further perpetuated by hostile attributions that are developed by both the parent and child about each other's intensions (Slep et al., 2018). For example, if a child assumes his mother intentionally assigns him a difficult chore to make him angry, and his mother assumes her child refuses to do the chore out of spite, both parties become increasingly dysregulated and more likely to engage in avoidance-based behaviors. Taken together, these mechanisms (i.e., emotional reactivity, cognitive errors, and behavioral avoidance) coalesce to form a mutually reinforcing coercive parent–child dynamic, which facilitates the escalation of negative and coercive behaviors that become entrenched and amplified over time. Thus, transdiagnostic interventions aimed at effectively treating pediatric irritability and disruptive behaviors must address underlying mechanisms existing at both individual and contextual levels.

Given its emphasis on transdiagnostic factors at both the child-focused and contextual levels, the Unified Protocol for the Transdiagnostic Treatment of Emotional Disorders in Children (UP-C) presents unique opportunities for effectively addressing factors hypothesized to maintain irritability and associated disruptive behaviors. As these symptoms tend to emerge in early childhood and are most responsive to treatment when addressed early on in a child's developmental trajectory (Fonagy & Luyten, 2018), initial efforts to develop a transdiagnostic treatment for pediatric irritability have been focused on modifying the UP-C, and not the Unified Protocol for the Transdiagnostic Treatment of Emotional Disorders in Adolescents (UP-A). Future research is necessary to determine if modifications can be made to the UP-A to effectively treat irritability in adolescents.

Figure 5.1 illustrates the hypothesized change process of this treatment model and highlights the desired shift in parent–child patterns of interaction during treatment. Namely, the parent–child dyad is initially shown engaging in negative emotional reactivity, attribution errors, and emotional behaviors (approach or avoidant), resulting in a coercive cycle that contributes to the development of disruptive behaviors in the child and ineffective parenting practices. In treatment,

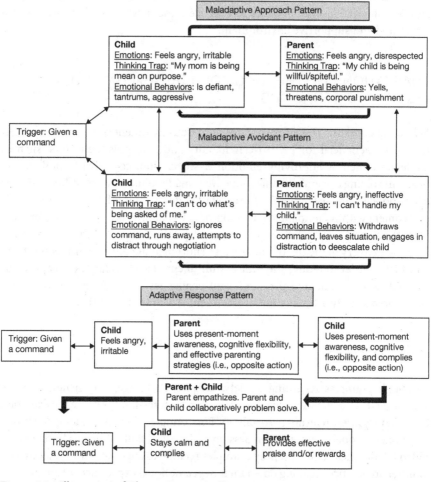

Figure 5.1. Illustration of Change Process in Treatment

the parent–child dyad is taught how to improve their emotional awareness, increase their cognitive flexibility, and engage in opposite action behaviors. These skills are reinforced in treatment through engagement in "frustration exposures." Through development and practice of these skills, the parent–child dyad works to remove themselves from this coercive interpersonal process and instead engage in a consistent, positive, and collaborative manner following participation in treatment.

As described in what follows, the group format of the UP-C for irritability supports parents and children in addressing this coercive interpersonal process by providing psychoeducation on emotions as well as behavioral and cognitive strategies aimed at extinguishing distress experienced during parent–child interactions that results in engagement in avoidance-based coping strategies. This education is provided in the respective parent and child groups, where they are also engaged in action-based learning activities, such as role plays, aimed at enhancing mastery of these techniques while in an emotionally regulated state. Parent–child dyads are then engaged in joint exposures aimed at heightening the child's emotional arousal in order to practice these newly learned strategies in a structured and supportive environment.

ADAPTATIONS OF THE UP-C FOR IRRITABILITY AND DISRUPTIVE BEHAVIORS

While the standard UP-C incorporates numerous treatment components thought to also be beneficial for pediatric irritability and disruptive behaviors, such as strategies aimed at improving emotion dysregulation, cognitive flexibility, and problem solving, several modifications were made to increase its utility with this client population (see Table 5.1 for a detailed description of each session's goals and content within the adapted curriculum for irritability, as well as key differences from the standard UP-C). Several of these adaptations impacted the overall structure and delivery of the treatment. We also shortened the number of sessions from 15 to 10 in order to reduce the time commitment placed on families, as previous research has documented the significant challenges with families of disruptive youth prematurely dropping out of treatment (Lavigne et al., 2010).

Child Curriculum

Although examples regarding anxiety, sadness, and anger are included in the standard UP-C, adaptations were made within each session to ensure the examples and role plays were relevant to irritability. For example, when introducing the three-component model of emotions in Session 2 of the "C" skill, clinicians initially provided hypothetical, child-friendly examples relating to anger, and then encouraged children to practice breaking down their own emotional experiences of anger, frustration, and/or irritability. In Session 3, rather than using an activation exercise

Table 5.1 OUTLINE OF TREATMENT PROTOCOL, PRIMARY SESSION GOALS, AND KEY DIFFERENCES FROM STANDARD UP-C

Session # (Skill)	Child Goals	Parent Goals	Joint Opposite Action or Exposure Activity	Key Differences from Standard UP-C
1 (C: Consider How I Feel)	Treatment structure/ rationale Behavioral contingencies	Treatment structure/rationale Three-component model of emotions Introduction to "Emotional Behavior" form (EBF)	Emotion identification Normalize emotions	More structured token system and behavioral expectations Earlier introduction of EBF
2 (C: Consider How I Feel)	Emotion identification and intensity rating Three-component model of emotions Cycle of emotional behaviors	Emotional and opposite parenting behaviors "Double Before, During, After" form Opposite parenting behavior: strategic attention	Collaborative reward identification	Enhanced discussion of role of approach behaviors in cycle of emotional behaviors Review EBF in parent group Revised opposite parenting behavior to "Strategic Attention"
3 (C: Consider How I Feel)	"Acting opposite" to emotional behaviors Emotion and behavior tracking	"Acting opposite" to emotional behaviors Psychoeducation about frustration tolerance exposure Opposite parenting behavior: consistency and reward systems Revise EBF	Opposite action exercise to practice frustration tolerance Parent coaching of strategic attention	In-session opposite action activity for frustration instead of sadness Changed "Emotion Thermometer for Happy" to "Emotion Thermometer for Calm, Relaxed, and Happy" Earlier introduction of present-moment awareness to parents Finalize EBF in parent group

Table 5.1 Continued

Session # (Skill)	Child Goals	Parent Goals	Joint Opposite Action or Exposure Activity	Key Differences from Standard UP-C
4 (C: Consider How I Feel)	Body clues/somatic awareness Body scanning Sensational exposure to body clues for anger/irritability	Body clues psychoeducation Body scanning Sensational exposure Opposite parenting behavior: expressing empathy	Opposite action exercise to practice frustration tolerance Parent coaching of selective attention and empathy	Enhanced emphasis on identifying body clues for anger Sensational exposures focused on body clues for anger Earlier introduction of opposite action/exposure exercises
5 (L: Look at My Thoughts)	Cognitive flexibility Psychoeducation Identify "thinking traps"	Cognitive flexibility and thinking traps Opposite parenting behavior: consistency and effective commands	Opposite action exercise to practice frustration tolerance Parent coaching of selective attention and empathy	Addition of "Out to Get Me Olaf" thinking trap Enhanced discussion of consistent use of effective commands/consequences Addition of opposite action/exposure exercise
6 (U: Use Detective Thinking and Problem Solving)	Introduction to detective thinking Detective thinking practice	Introduction to detective thinking and cognitive flexibility Opposite parenting behavior: consistency and effective punishment procedures	Opposite action exercise to practice frustration tolerance Parent coaching of opposite parenting behaviors	Emphasis on "Out to Get Me Olaf" for detective thinking More extensive discussion of consistency and effective punishment procedures Addition of opposite action/exposure exercise
7 (U: Use Detective Thinking and Problem Solving)	Introduction to problem solving Problem-solving practice	Introduction to problem solving Shaping and supporting problem-solving practice at home Opposite parenting behavior: healthy independence granting	Parent–child problem-solving practice Parent coaching to reinforce problem solving and expressing empathy	Enhanced focus on problem solving in situations that elicit anger, aggression, etc. Use of hot-headed and cool-headed descriptors to evaluate solutions Enhanced parent coaching during problem-solving practice

Session				
8 (E: Experience My Feelings)	Introduction to present-moment awareness Present-moment awareness practice Awareness of emotions	Introduction to present-moment awareness Introduction to exposure Opposite parenting behavior: healthy and helpful modeling of emotions	Opposite action exercise to practice frustration tolerance Parent coaching of opposite parenting behaviors	Practice present-moment awareness after frustration induction in child group Earlier introduction to exposure in parent group Addition of opposite action/exposure exercise
9 (E: Experience My Feelings)	Rationale for exposure Demonstration and execution of situational emotion exposure Individual/small-group exposures	Review of exposures and opposite parenting behaviors	Parent–child exposure practice, with therapist coaching	Only one session devoted explicitly to exposure Exposures focused on anger/frustration/irritability Enhanced parent coaching during exposures
10 (S: Stay Healthy and Happy)	Skills review Plan for facing strong emotions in future	Skills review Plan to support child in facing strong emotions	Celebration of progress	None

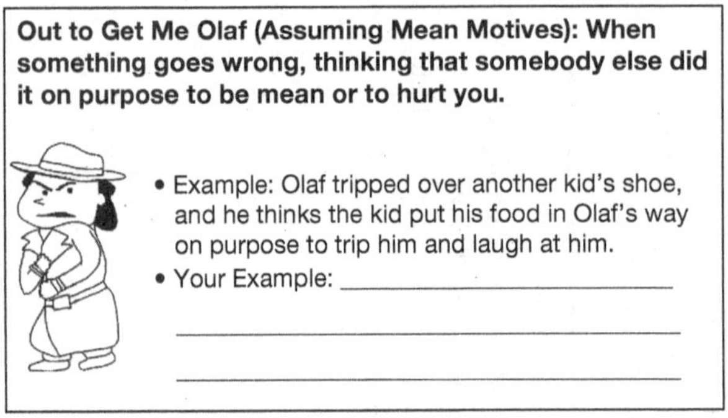

> **Out to Get Me Olaf (Assuming Mean Motives): When something goes wrong, thinking that somebody else did it on purpose to be mean or to hurt you.**
>
> - Example: Olaf tripped over another kid's shoe, and he thinks the kid put his food in Olaf's way on purpose to trip him and laugh at him.
> - Your Example: _____
>   _____
>   _____

Figure 5.2. "Out to Get Me Olaf" Thinking Trap Character

to practice acting opposite to sadness, clinicians introduced the concept of acting opposite by having the children engage in a mild frustration-inducing exposure, and then encouraging them to engage in an activity to practice acting opposite to frustration or irritability. Similarly, sensational exposures in Session 4 focused on eliciting physiological sensations associated with frustration or irritability (e.g., wall sits to elicit muscle tension, use of heating pads to elicit temperature changes). During the "U" stage of treatment, in which strategies are taught regarding cognitive flexibility and problem solving, several modifications were made to address unique cognitive aspects of irritability. For example, an additional thinking trap (i.e., "Out to Get Me Olaf" or "assuming mean motives") was included to explicitly address the hostile attribution bias commonly noted in irritable and/or disruptive youth (see Figure 5.2). Furthermore, when discussing problem solving, additional coaching was provided regarding how to appropriately evaluate the "pros" and "cons" for each solution identified. More specifically, children were taught to distinguish between "hot-headed" solutions (ones that may get them into trouble and/or hurt relationships with others) and "cool-headed" solutions (ones that will keep them out of trouble and preserve relationships with others) to further refine insight into behavioral consequences and perspective-taking abilities. Throughout the child curriculum, reduced emphasis was placed on the use of worksheets included in the standard UP-C, since this client population often has more difficulty sustaining attention (Brotman et al., 2017; U.S. Department of Education, 2008). Instead, psychoeducation regarding the various topics in the manual was largely demonstrated through action-based learning activities (e.g., group-based whiteboard discussions, games, modeling by therapists, role plays).

Parent Curriculum

Although the standard UP-C curriculum includes a strong parent component, modifications were made to centralize the importance of parent management strategies. Strategies included and emphasized are based on Kaminski et al.'s

(2008) meta-analysis that highlighted the treatment components most predictive of positive outcomes with disruptive and/or irritable youth. These included parents engaging in positive interactions with their child, responding consistently to problematic behaviors, utilizing effective command-punishment procedures, and modeling healthy emotional coping. The traditional UP-C framework of "emotional parenting" and "opposite parenting" behaviors was retained, as were the four emotional parenting behaviors (overcontrol/overprotection, criticism, inconsistency, and excessive emotional modeling). However, the emotional parenting behaviors were modified to reflect how they manifest with an irritable child, and opposite parenting behaviors were enhanced to provide more robust parent management strategies for children with disruptive behaviors. For example, while discussing overcontrol/overprotection, emphasis was placed on reducing psychological control practices commonly used by parents of irritable youth and instead using collaborative parenting approaches to promote their child's independence, compliance, and problem-solving abilities. Discussions of overcontrol/overprotection also focused on assisting parents in recognizing how avoidance of activities and situations in which their child may display irritable or dysregulated behavior may be negatively reinforcing to the parent in the short term but may perpetuate child avoidance and distress intolerance in the longer term. Consistent with the standard UP-C, parents were taught the information discussed in the child group, but increased emphasis was placed on how to collaboratively support their child in practicing and using these strategies through parent management techniques.

Joint Opposite Action and Exposure Activities

We structured each 90-minute group treatment session to include at least 20 to 30 minutes of joint parent–child experiential activities (i.e., acting opposite and/or exposures) each week. Many of these activities involved exposure to frustration or anger-inducing stimuli, ranging from being asked to complete a very difficult puzzle within a time limit to having a conversation with their parent about an ongoing conflict at home. Chosen activities were often based on items from the "Emotional Behavior" form (see Figure 5.3 for an example), which parents and children were asked to begin creating in the first several sessions, in contrast with its later presentation in standard UP-C. During these joint opposite action and exposure activities, the parent–child dyads were supported in practicing the various child-focused and parent-focused skills they learned in their respective groups and were provided with coaching from therapy providers. These dyadic, exposure-based exercises are viewed as a critical component of this adapted UP-C curriculum, particularly considering the results from a meta-analysis examining the efficacy of parent management training (PMT) that showed in-session dyadic skills practice to be predictive of better treatment outcomes (Kaminski et al., 2008).

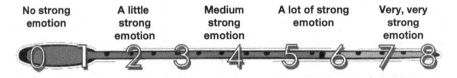

Situation	Emotional Behavior	How strong is the emotion (0-8)?	Did you work on it (Y/N)?
Told to stop playing video games	Screamed, cried, threw controller	8	N
Doing math homework	Avoided it, didn't finish it	7	Y
Teased by a student at recess	Punched, kicked another student	7	N
Told to take a shower	Hid in room and played on tablet	6	N
Lost a board game	Threw game pieces, accused others of cheating	5	Y
Taking a test	Doodled on paper, didn't answer several questions	4	N
Fighting with brother over preferred TV show	Hid the remote, called brother names	3	Y
Completing chores	Ignored mom, ran outside to play	3	Y
Told to make his bed	Lied and said it was done	2	N
Told to brush his teeth	Pretended to brush them	2	Y

Figure 5.3. Example of a Completed "Emotional Behavior" Form

EVIDENCE-BASED INTERVENTIONS FOR IRRITABILITY AND DISRUPTIVE BEHAVIORS

Two groups of interventions are typically utilized to treat disruptive behavior disorders: PMT and child-focused cognitive-behavioral therapy (CBT; Kaminski & Claussen, 2017). PMT intends to disrupt parent–child coercive cycles that maintain disruptive behaviors by helping parents learn new parenting strategies (e.g., providing praise, consistent responses to behavioral concerns; Patterson, 1982). In contrast, child-focused CBT interventions focus on improving individual-level deficits in areas of emotion regulation, cognitive appraisal, and social skills (e.g., Lochman et al., 2008; Sukhodolsky et al., 2016).

Several emerging treatments have shown some initial promise in addressing irritability in youth. The Modular Approach to Therapy for Children (MATCH; Chorpita & Weisz, 2009), which includes common elements taken from PMT and CBT, is a modular, transdiagnostic approach that has been shown to be efficacious in treating disruptive behaviors and has some preliminary support for treating irritability in youth (Evans, 2020). Another emerging approach to treating irritability in youth is focused on combining PMT interventions and exposure-based strategies for tolerating and managing frustration (Kircanski et al., 2019), although empirical results of this approach are still forthcoming.

Despite emerging research on irritability as a transdiagnostic construct, and the development of new irritability-focused treatments cited earlier, diagnostic status continues to dictate practice guidelines. Per the most recent evidence-based update for disruptive behavior disorders, PMT is the only well-established treatment, while child-focused CBT is classified as probably efficacious (Kaminski & Claussen, 2017). Therefore, when treating irritability in youth with a primary disruptive behavior disorder or attention-deficit/hyperactivity disorder (ADHD), PMT is likely to continue to be the first-line recommended approach. UP-C for irritability would be a reasonable alternative to PMT for youth presenting with comorbid internalizing/externalizing disorders or for youth with disruptive mood dysregulation disorder, for which an evidence base is still emerging.

EMPIRICAL SUPPORT FOR THE USE OF THE UP-C WITH IRRITABILITY AND DISRUPTIVE BEHAVIORS

The adapted version of UP-C for irritability and disruptive behaviors was evaluated within a retrospective study that provided promising initial support for the feasibility and acceptability of the modified UP-C in the treatment of pediatric irritability (Hawks et al., 2020). Attrition rates for families that received this intervention were lower than those typically seen for this client population (Lavigne et al., 2010). The majority of parents reported they were able to understand and use the information presented in group and that they intended to continue using the strategies discussed. Furthermore, parents reported high satisfaction following participation in this group-based treatment. This was particularly noteworthy given the emphasis placed on opposite action/exposure-based exercises, as both children and parents frequently became emotionally activated during these joint activities. High therapist adherence to the intervention also supported the feasibility of the modified UP-C.

Although the sample size of this study was small ($n = 19$) and power was limited to detect significant effects, several initial efficacy results appeared promising in favor of this modified UP-C for anger and irritability. Perhaps most notably, parents' reports of their child's irritability significantly decreased from pre- to post-treatment. Similarly, parents reported a significant reduction in their child's overall engagement in oppositional behaviors across the course of treatment. Mild improvements in their child's engagement in prosocial behaviors were also reported by parents. On a measure assessing overall child difficulties, including both emotional and behavioral problems, parents reported a significant decrease from pre- to post-treatment. This is a particularly critical finding, as previous studies have demonstrated that improving parents' perceptions of their child's disruptive behaviors can result in improved use of effective and consistent parenting practices, thereby reducing their engagement in coercive processes (Slep et al., 2018).

APPLICATION OF THE UP-C TO IRRITABILITY AND DISRUPTIVE BEHAVIORS: A CASE EXAMPLE

This case example illustrates a typical course of treatment for a client and parent participating in group-based therapy utilizing the UP-C adapted for irritability and disruptive behaviors.

Case Description

"Brandon" was a 10-year-old, multiracial male who presented for treatment with co-principal diagnoses of disruptive mood dysregulation disorder and ADHD, combined presentation. Brandon's mother described him as "always being difficult." She noted that he was constantly irritable and quick to anger. Brandon reported that he often gets in trouble at home/school and described many of these situations as "unfair" and stated that others were purposely trying to get him into trouble. Brandon's mother reported they have tried "everything" and "consequences don't work with him." Brandon and his mother were referred to participate in the adapted UP-C outpatient multi-family group due to these concerns.

Intervention

Brandon and his mother participated in all 10 sessions of the group-based treatment. Brandon was taught to identify strong emotions and emotional behaviors and then practiced acting opposite to these tendencies through use of approach-based behaviors and cognitive flexibility. For example, Brandon was taught to recognize his "Out to Get Me Olaf" thinking trap thoughts related to peers (e.g., "That kid bumped into me in the hallway on purpose") and then learned ways to use his detective thinking to reappraise these thoughts (e.g., "The hallways are really crowded. I'm sure that kid bumped into me by accident").

Brandon's mother was taught the material learned in the child group to help her support Brandon in generalizing the skills outside of therapy sessions. She was also taught about common emotional parenting behaviors and how to act opposite to these tendencies by using effective behavior management strategies. For example, she was taught how to recognize when she was being inconsistent in her use of praise, effective commands, or consequences (i.e., emotional parenting) and how to be more consistent in use of these strategies (i.e., acting opposite).

Brandon and his mother participated in weekly parent–child "frustration exposures" during Sessions 3 through 9. The content of these exposures was derived from the "Emotional Behavior" form (see Figure 5.3) completed by Brandon and his mother during Session 1. Prior to beginning exposures, Brandon was introduced to the concept of engaging in a "science experiment" to see what would happen if he acted opposite to frustration or anger (e.g., by expressing feelings in a calm voice when angry rather than throwing something). He participated in a group frustration exposure in session with the other children, during which the children practiced acting opposite when exposed to a mildly frustrating stimulus (e.g., listening to an annoying noise for two minutes). Clinicians obtained frustration ratings before, during, and after the exposure and drew the attention of the children to changes in their frustration over time and ways in which they were able to manage the frustration in a helpful and prosocial manner. After being introduced to exposures as "acting opposite" experiments, Brandon and his mother began participating in exposures together at the end of Session 3. During these joint frustration exposures, Brandon was intentionally exposed to a stimulus or situation from his hierarchy likely to elicit frustration. During the exposure, Brandon and his mother were encouraged to practice using skills learned in session with each other, while receiving modeling and coaching from the group therapists. For example, in Session 9, Brandon and his mother participated in a frustration exposure related to his difficulty completing his math homework. Brandon's mother brought a math homework sheet to session and prompted Brandon to complete it during the exposure. Initially, Brandon became quite frustrated and engaged in several emotional behaviors aimed at avoiding the task (e.g., scribbling on the worksheet, negotiating, arguing). The clinician working with Brandon and his mother encouraged him to engage in opposite action, while also coaching Brandon's mother in effective use of opposite action parenting behaviors. As a result, Brandon's mother was able to prompt Brandon to engage in opposite action through her use of an effective command–consequence sequence. With these prompts, Brandon was able to complete the worksheet and was praised for his efforts by his mom and the group therapist.

The following script illustrates the parent–child interactions, as well as clinician coaching, that occurred during this frustration exposure:

Mother: *Brandon, please pick up your pencil and begin working on your math homework.*

Brandon: *I hate math! Why couldn't you pick something easier for me to do?! Can't I do some English homework instead?! (Starts scribbling on the worksheet and crumpling it up)*

Mother: *Brandon, please pick up your pencil and begin working on your math homework or you will lose screen time for the rest of the night. And stop scribbling all over that worksheet and crumpling it up; you're going to ruin it!*

Clinician: *Mom, you're doing a great job sticking with the command–consequence sequence. Remember, try to also ignore any of those emotional behaviors Brandon might be engaging in right now, like the scribbling or negotiating. Brandon, I know you're feeling super frustrated right now, which means it would be a great time to try engaging in some "opposite action" behaviors like we've been practicing! Remember, if you can stick with it, you'll be able to earn all your points for today!*

Brandon: *Ugh! Fine, I'll do it, but I still think this is stupid! (Begins to pick up his pencil and look at the math homework)*

Mother: *Brandon, I am so proud of you for getting started on your math homework!!! (Continues to ignore any emotional behaviors, such as calling the exposure "stupid")*

Clinician: *Nice job, mom! Way to praise him for engaging in those opposite action behaviors! Brandon, so impressed by your decision to engage in some opposite action and get started on that worksheet!*

POTENTIAL BARRIERS AND TROUBLESHOOTING

Given that both PMT and exposure-based interventions for tolerating and managing strong emotions have been hypothesized as key elements in the treatment of pediatric irritability (Stringaris et al., 2018), successful use of opposite action/exposure-based exercises is a critical component of this intervention. However, despite its importance, it can be difficult to successfully complete frustration exposures with this client population. Often parents will respond with strong negative emotions when informed that they are going to intentionally induce frustration in their child during group sessions. This is not altogether surprising, given the previously described coercive cycle. Thus, it is very important to thoroughly explain the rationale for and process of engaging in these exposures over the course of treatment (i.e., remove parent–child dyad from coercive cycle, encourage use of effective strategies for coping with strong emotions). Clinicians should emphasize that these frustration exposures are intended to evoke strong emotions in both the parent and child to allow both parties to practice using the strategies they are learning in their respective groups. Parents will frequently express fears that their child might exhibit significant behavioral concerns during frustration exposures. Therapists should be sure to describe how graduated exposures will work and note that they will be there to provide support.

Similarly, children may be resistant to the idea of participating in activities that will frustrate them and then be expected to "act opposite," as they have typically been previously negatively reinforced for engaging in emotional behaviors during frustrating experiences. Therapists should be sure to explain the rationale for engaging in these exposures, establish clear expectations, and provide consistent consequences. Children will be more likely to engage in opposite action/prosocial behaviors if pre-established rewards are available contingent on their behavior during exposures. Thus, it is recommended that a reward system be used throughout the group curriculum to enhance motivation to engage in didactic and experiential activities.

Finally, therapists may also be reluctant to engage clients and parents in frustration exposures due to the fear that they will be unable to manage any significant behavioral outbursts. When training new clinicians in the use of frustration exposures, it is critical that they understand the rationale for these activities and can articulate this rationale to children and parents. Specifically, the therapist should emphasize that the purpose of exposing the child to triggers for frustration is to improve the child's ability to tolerate uncomfortable emotions and learn that they are capable of using skills to act opposite to strong emotions rather than engaging in unhelpful, inappropriate, or aggressive behaviors. Skills practice and exposure should be integrated when using UP-C to address irritability, as practice of new behaviors in session is crucial for helping youth overcome the tendency to engage in inappropriate or unhelpful emotional behaviors. Children may benefit from engaging in problem solving prior to exposures to identify ways they will practice acting opposite when frustrated, or from generating a coping thought they will use if they start to fall into the "Out to Get Me Olaf" thinking trap. This integration of skills and exposure is crucial, as anecdotally parents of irritable children often complain that although their child appears to understand and is even able to practice a skill when calm, they struggle or are unwilling to implement skills when escalated, and parents in turn struggle during these times with effectively prompting skills use or managing behavior. The importance of constructing appropriate exposures should be discussed. Therapists should be well versed in the use of behavior management strategies, such as strategic attention and contingent consequences, and know how to effectively use these strategies during a frustration exposure. They should feel comfortable modeling and coaching parents in how to support their child through an exposure. In order to develop comfort and mastery of this intervention, therapists should be provided with ample opportunities to practice engaging in exposures prior to working with families.

Tip Sheet for Using UP-C in Youth with Anger/Irritability/Disruptive Behaviors

✓ **Why use UP-C for anger/irritability/disruptive behaviors?**
- UP-C can address:
  - High negative emotionality
  - Oppositional behaviors
  - Ineffective parenting practices (e.g., inconsistency, harsh or permissive parenting)
  - Low parental confidence and distress tolerance.

✓ **How do I use UP-C for anger/irritability/disruptive behaviors?**
- Use fewer worksheets. Instead, use active tasks, role plays, and therapist modeling.
- Utilize more behavior management strategies, including:
  - Strategic attention
  - Effective commands
  - Frequent reinforcement
  - Consistent consequences
- Increase focus of parental intervention on:
  - Promoting positive interactions (i.e., reduce criticism)
  - Consistency in responses to problematic behaviors
  - Modeling healthy emotional coaching
- Use the hostile attribution bias thinking trap ("Out to Get Me Olaf") to promote cognitive flexibility.
- Encourage insight into consequences of actions when teaching problem solving.
- Use frustration exposures early and often with parent–child dyads.
  - Emphasize collaboratively practicing parent and child skills with active coaching from therapists.

✓ **What challenges might come up when using UP-C for anger/ irritability/disruptive behaviors?**
- Youth may quickly become bored and disengaged during group discussions.
  - Be sure to provide frequent positive reinforcement and use activities whenever possible to illustrate concepts.
- Youth may become dysregulated and exhibit disruptive behaviors during exposures.
  - Initially, make sure to choose mild opposite action experiments and use effective behavior management strategies throughout.
- Parents may struggle to effectively apply behavior management strategies and become emotionally dysregulated during exposures.
  - Therapists will need to provide modeling and coaching to parents when this occurs. Praising parents for demonstrating skills is helpful.

✓ **When is UP-C not appropriate for angry/irritable/disruptive youth?**
- If a child is engaging in significant conduct problems resulting in harm to self or others, or is involved in the criminal justice system, a more intensive treatment option such as multisystemic therapy may be appropriate.

REFERENCES

American Psychiatric Association. (2013). *Diagnostic and statistical manual of mental disorders* (5th ed.). American Psychiatric Publishing.

Brotman, M. A., Kircanski, K., & Leibenluft, E. (2017). Irritability in children and adolescents. *Annual Review of Clinical Psychology, 13*, 317–341.

Brotman, M. A., Schmajuk, M., Rich, B. A., Dickstein, D. P., Guyer, A. E., Costello, E. J., Egger, H. L., Angold, A., Pine, D. S., & Leibenluft, E. (2006). Prevalence, clinical correlates, and longitudinal course of severe mood dysregulation in children. *Biological Psychiatry, 60*, 991–997.

Ehrenreich-May, J., & Chu, B. C. (2014). *Transdiagnostic treatments for children and adolescents: Principles and practice.* Guilford Press.

Eisenberg, N., Cumberland, A., Spinrad, T. L., Fabes, R. A., Shepard, S. A., Reiser, M., Murphy, B. C., Losoya, S. H., & Guthrie, I. K. (2001). The relations of regulation and emotionality to children's externalizing and internalizing problem behavior. *Child Development, 72*, 1112–1134.

Evans, S. C., Burke, J. D., Roberts, M. C., Fite, P. J., Lochman, J. E., Francisco, R., & Reed, G. M. (2017). Irritability in child and adolescent psychopathology: An integrative review for ICD-11. *Clinical Psychology Review, 53*, 29–45.

Evans, S., Weisz, J., Carvalho, A., Garibaldi, P., Bearman, S., & Chorpita, B. (2020). Effects of standard and modular psychotherapies in the treatment of youth with severe irritability. *Journal of Consulting and Clinical Psychology, 88*(3), 255–268.

Fonagy, P., & Luyten, P. (2018). Conduct problems in youth and the RDoC approach: A developmental, evolutionary-based view. *Clinical Psychology Review, 64*, 57–76.

Hawks, J. L., Kennedy, S. M., Holzman, J. B. W., & Ehrenreich-May, J. (2020). Development and application of an innovative transdiagnostic treatment approach for pediatric irritability. *Behavior Therapy, 51*(2), 334–349.

Kaminski, J. W., & Claussen, A. H. (2017). Evidence base update for psychosocial treatments for disruptive behaviors in children. *Journal of Clinical Child & Adolescent Psychology, 46*(4), 477–499.

Kaminski, J. W., Valle, L. A., Filene, J. H., & Boyle, C. L. (2008). A meta-analytic review of components associated with parent training effectiveness. *Journal of Abnormal Child Psychology, 36*, 567–589.

Kircanski, K., Craske, M., Averbeck, B., Pine, D., Leibenluft, E., & Brotman, M. (2019). Exposure therapy for pediatric irritability: Theory and potential mechanisms. *Behaviour Research and Therapy, 118*, 141–149.

Kolko, D., Dorn, L., Bukstein, O., & Burke, J. (2008). Clinically referred ODD children with or without CD and healthy controls: Comparisons across contextual domains. *Journal of Family Studies, 17*, 714–734.

Lavigne, J. V., LeBailly, S. A., Gouze, K. R., Binns, H. J., Keller, J., & Pate, L. (2010). Predictors and correlates of completing behavioral parent training for the treatment of oppositional defiant disorder. *Behavior Therapy, 41*(2), 198–211.

Lochman, J. E., Wells, K., & Lenhart, L. A. (2008). *Coping Power: Child group facilitator's guide* (Vol. 2). Oxford University Press.

Moore, A. A., Lapato, D. M., Brotman, M. A., Leibenluft, E., Aggen, S. H., Hettema, J. M., York, T. P., Silberg, J. L., & Roberson-Nay, R. (2019). Heritability, stability, and prevalence of tonic and phasic irritability as indicators of disruptive mood dysregulation disorder. *Journal of Child Psychology and Psychiatry, 60,* 1032–1041.

Nolen-Hoeksema, S., & Watkins, E. R. (2011). A heuristic for developing transdiagnostic models of psychopathology: Explaining multifinality and divergent trajectories. *Perspectives on Psychological Science, 6*(6), 589–609.

Patterson, G. R. (1982). *Coercive family process* (Vol. 3). Castalia Publishing Company.

Reid, S. C., Salmon, K., & Lovibond, P. F. (2006). Cognitive biases in childhood anxiety, depression, and aggression: Are they pervasive or specific? *Cognitive Therapy and Research, 30*(5), 531–549.

Slep, A. M., Heyman, R. E., Mitnick, D. M., Lorber, M. F., & Beauchaine, T. P. (2018). Targeting couple and parent-child coercion to improve health behaviors. *Behavior Research and Therapy, 101,* 82–91.

Sukhodolsky, D. G., Smith, S. D., McCauley, S. A., Ibrahim, K., & Piasecka, J. B. (2016). Behavioral interventions for anger, irritability, and aggression in children and adolescents. *Journal of Child and Adolescent Psychopharmacology, 26,* 58–64.

U.S. Department of Education, Office of Special Education and Rehabilitative Services, Office of Special Education Programs. (2008). *Teaching children with attention deficit hyperactivity disorder: Instructional strategies and practices.*

6

The Unified Protocol for Use with Adolescents with or at Risk for Serious Mental Illness

MARC J. WEINTRAUB AND JAMIE ZINBERG ■

In this chapter, serious mental illness (SMI) refers to psychotic disorders (most commonly schizophrenia) and bipolar disorder. SMI affects about 5% to 6% of the population, with an average age of onset in the early to mid-20s (Kessler et al., 2005a). These conditions are increasingly conceptualized as neurodevelopmental disorders, as the first clinical manifestations become evident years prior to the onset of SMI. Based on retrospective recall from individuals who have developed a SMI, the first emergence of symptoms typically occurs 10 years or more before onset of the full-threshold disorder (Shaw et al., 2005). As a result, 50% to 65% of individuals who develop an SMI show their first symptoms in adolescence (Kessler et al., 2005b). These "early rumblings" of SMI symptoms phenotypically are similar to the full-threshold symptom presentations but are less severe and/or shorter in duration. Alongside early mood difficulties and/or psychotic experiences, functional declines commonly emerge in social, academic/occupational, and cognitive domains.

PSYCHOSIS RISK SYNDROMES

The evolution of the prodromal (i.e., forerunning) period of SMI is illustrated in Figure 6.1. While there is no official diagnosis in the *Diagnostic and Statistical Manual of Mental Disorders* for the psychosis risk syndromes, the DSM-5 does outline criteria for the attenuated psychosis syndrome under "Conditions for Further Study." These symptoms include the presence of mild positive symptoms (i.e., unusual thought content/delusions, suspiciousness, grandiosity, and/or

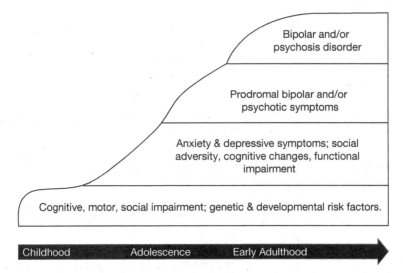

Figure 6.1. The Evolution of Symptoms and Risk Factors in the Development of Psychosis Recreated from figure presented in Howes & Murray, 2014.

perceptual abnormalities/hallucinations); the symptoms must be present at least once per week over the last month and they must have begun within the past year (American Psychiatric Association, 2013). Although many of these individuals have symptoms of psychosis (e.g., hearing whispers or seeing shadows), they are not fully convinced in their beliefs/experiences and the symptoms do not meet threshold for a full psychotic-spectrum disorder.

The attenuated psychosis syndrome accounts for about 80% to 90% of individuals who meet criteria for psychosis risk (Woods et al., 2009). There are two other psychosis risk syndromes that are considerably less common. Genetic risk with recent deterioration syndrome includes individuals who have a first-degree relative with any psychotic disorder and a 30% (or greater) drop in their Global Assessment of Functioning (GAF) score over the past year. Criteria for the final psychosis risk syndrome, brief intermittent psychosis syndrome, are met if the person experiences any psychotic-intensity symptoms (i.e., the client had full conviction that the experiences were real) and the experiences began in the past three months and were present for at least several minutes a day at a frequency of at least once per month. However, to meet criteria for this risk syndrome, a current psychotic disorder must be ruled out by insufficient frequency, duration, or "urgency" (e.g., client didn't require hospitalization) to meet criteria for a psychotic disorder (McGlashan et al., 2001).

RISK FOR BIPOLAR DISORDER

The prodromal phases of bipolar disorder have received comparatively less research attention than prodromal psychosis. Nonetheless, there are evidence-based operational definitions to identify individuals who are at high-risk status for the disorder. Individuals are deemed high risk for bipolar disorder if they experience subsyndromal hypomanic symptoms and major depressive episode(s). Researchers have most commonly used a modified version of DSM-5's unspecified bipolar disorder to determine if a client meets criteria for subsyndromal hypomania (Birmaher et al., 2009); these criteria include distinct periods of elevated, expansive, or irritable mood plus two (three, if irritable only) DSM symptoms of hypomania. Symptoms must cause a change in functioning for at least four hours per day and must be present for 10 days or more in the individual's lifetime, but the symptoms do not meet full criteria for bipolar I or II disorder. Of note, risk is increased if the client has a first- or second- degree relative with bipolar disorder, as a family loading of bipolar disorder is the single most predictive risk factor the development of the disorder (Axelson et al., 2015).

TREATMENT IMPLICATIONS

The early stages of SMI in youth and adolescents are a critical period for treatment, as delays in treatment or undertreatment are associated with longer and more severe courses of illness, higher likelihood of remission, increased need for hospitalization, and poorer functioning (Birmaher et al., 2014; Weintraub et al., 2020a). Unfortunately, fewer than half of individuals with SMI symptoms receive mental health care in a given year. Further, only about 15% of those individuals who receive care are fortunate enough to receive evidence-based treatment (Wang et al., 2005). One of the reasons that so many SMI clients go untreated is that they are excluded from many general clinical programs. Clinicians often report feeling underprepared and/or unwilling to treat SMI, which leaves many of these treatment-seeking individuals taking whatever mental health care they can find (Humphreys, 2017).

HOW THE UNIFIED PROTOCOL APPLIES TO SMI

Meeting criteria for a risk diagnosis does not mean that the client will go on to develop the disorder for which they are deemed at risk. The conversion rate from a psychosis risk syndrome to a full-threshold psychotic disorder is about 36% over a three-year period, and the rate of conversion to bipolar I or II disorder from a high-risk classification is about 15% to 45% over a period of one to 4.5 years (Axelson et al., 2015; Fusar-Poli et al., 2012). In addition to SMI symptoms, the vast majority of individuals with or at risk for SMI have comorbid emotional (mood and/or anxiety) disorders that precede and co-occur with their SMI symptoms. In individuals with psychotic symptoms, upwards of 70% have an emotional disorder (Addington et al., 2017). Of this 70%, 50% have an anxiety disorder and 60% have a depressive disorder. Adolescents with bipolar spectrum conditions almost always have had a history of major depression. Additionally, between 25% and 50% have a secondary anxiety disorder diagnosis (Duffy et al., 2013; Weintraub et al., 2020b). Thus, the clinical picture for individuals with SMI is symptomatically heterogeneous, with a combination of mood, anxiety, manic, and psychotic symptoms.

One of the primary justifications put forth for the development of the Unified Protocol (UP) is that comorbidities between emotional disorders reflect overlapping psychological processes between disorders, including cognitive, behavioral, and emotional dysfunction (Brown & Barlow, 2009). The same underlying processes that underlie emotional disorders are also present in SMI. Emotional dysregulation, greater emotional reactivity, and increased experiences of negative emotions are present in emotional disorders and are also fundamental disruptions in individuals with SMI (Green et al., 2007; Sloan et al., 2017). Negative cognitions and maladaptive thinking styles are thought to play both a causal and maintaining role across each of these disorders (Beck & Haigh, 2014). Finally, behavioral dysfunction, including avoidance behaviors, social withdrawal and isolation, and emotional tantrums/fights with others, is a common response and reinforcer to emotional and SMI symptoms. As in emotional disorder, these common underlying cognitive, behavioral, and emotional difficulties have led to the development of disorder-specific cognitive-behavioral therapy (CBT). Unsurprisingly, CBT has been found to be efficacious in treating mood and psychotic symptoms in individuals with SMI (Hutton & Taylor, 2014; West et al., 2017).

Due to the varied psychiatric presentations and the overlapping psychological processes between these varied presentations (as well as the uncertain clinical outcomes of youth at risk for SMI), many SMI experts have proposed turning away from disorder-specific psychosocial treatments and focusing on broader symptoms and skills when treating individuals at risk for SMI (McGorry & Nelson, 2016). To that end, the Unified Protocol for Transdiagnostic Treatment of Emotional Disorders in Adolescents (UP-A) appears to be an ideal fit, as it focuses on broad symptoms and skills that are fundamental to the cognitive, behavioral, and emotional difficulties that are present across these conditions.

DELIVERY OF THE UP-A TO ADOLESCENTS WITH SMI SYMPTOMS

We have been delivering the UP-A in a group treatment format at the UCLA Jane and Terry Semel Institute for Neuroscience and Human Behavior since 2018. Prior to providing this service, the UP-A lacked an evidence base for individuals with SMI symptoms. Thus, we became interested in testing the treatment's acceptability and efficacy in improving psychiatric symptoms and functioning with youth who have begun to experience subsyndromal, yet distressing, symptoms of bipolar mood and/or psychotic symptoms.

The typical flow of the group treatment for adolescents with SMI symptoms shown in Table 6.1. All of the UP-A protocol was maintained; however, we made a couple of additions to the protocol as follows. First, in the "Emotion Identification

Table 6.1 SESSION-BY-SESSION SUMMARY OF THE UP-A WITH SMI SYMPTOMS

Session	Title	Session Content
1	Building and Keeping Motivation	• Build rapport with adolescents. • Discuss key problems and set goals. • Determine what motivates the adolescents to change.
2	Emotion Identification Practice; Getting to Know Your Emotions	• Provide psychoeducation about different emotions. • Discuss the purpose of emotions. • Develop the adolescents' awareness of their feelings. • Teach "I" statements to communicate emotions.
3	Linking Emotions to Thoughts & Behaviors	• Introduce the three parts of an emotion. • Introduce the cycle of avoidance and other emotional behaviors. • Introduce some common thinking traps (i.e., cognitive distortions). • Teach the adolescents how to track emotions, thoughts, and behaviors.
4 & 5	Being Flexible in Your Thinking	• Review common thinking traps (i.e., cognitive distortions). • Develop the adolescents' ability to think flexibly about emotional situations. • Link thoughts to actions by teaching detective thinking and problem-solving skills.
6	Awareness of Emotional Experiences	• Introduce and practice present-moment awareness. • Introduce and practice nonjudgmental awareness. • Compare and contrast detective thinking and mindful awareness.
7 & 8	Introduction to Emotion-Focused Behavioral Experiments & Situational Emotion Exposure	• Introduce the concepts of opposite action and emotion-focused behavioral experiments. • Discuss the rationale for situational emotion exposures, introduced to the adolescents as another type of behavioral experiment. • Conduct sensational exposure exercises to help the adolescents learn to tolerate uncomfortable physical feelings. • Brainstorm situational emotion exposures in session and assign exposures for home learning. • Engage the adolescents in emotion-focused behavioral experiments for sadness, anxiety, and other emotions.
9	Reviewing Accomplishments and Looking Ahead	• Review skills and progress toward goals. • Create a relapse prevention plan.

Practice" and "Getting to Know Your Emotions" exercises, the adolescents are taught a method of communicating emotions using "I" statements. This was added to increase awareness of their emotions as well as to facilitate communication between adolescents and their parent(s). For example, a teen who is anxious/suspicious of public places could communicate, "When I go into town, I feel nervous and mistrustful of others." Second, the flexible thinking and cognitive reappraisal (UP-A Module 5) and the present-moment awareness and nonjudgmental awareness sessions (UP-A Module 6) are conducted prior to the behavioral experiments and situational exposures. We reordered these modules for this population because (1) cognitive distortions can be more acutely distressing for adolescents with SMI symptoms than their behaviors, (2) not all of the participants have identifiable problematic avoidance behaviors (e.g., an adolescent at risk for bipolar disorder who experiences irritability and grandiosity may have problems with approach behaviors as opposed to avoidance), and (3) we found it to be helpful (and occasionally necessary) for many of these adolescents to have cognitive tools (e.g., cognitive reappraisal) when engaging with behavioral experiments and exposures. Of note, for teens who cannot identify avoidance behaviors when we begin the situational exposures, we ask them to identify any problem behavior (e.g., angrily yelling at their parents) and devise an emotion ladder for engaging in opposite action related to that problem behavior.

We also teach participants deep breathing (termed diaphragmatic breathing) in the first five sessions and then a mindful breathing space meditation for the final four sessions (coinciding with the presentation of Module 6 and then also paired with the behavioral experiments and situational exposures). Given that most of the adolescents experienced distressing emotions, these exercises were implemented as a way to provide the them with additional methods to manage their stress.

A final addition is the inclusion of SMI-specific experiences as examples throughout the emotional awareness and detective thinking modules. Emotions and thoughts relating to experiences like suspiciousness, grandiosity, confusion, ideas of reference, and elevated mood are discussed. Having the group leader provide examples has seemed to reduce the stigma of these experiences and increases the likelihood that the adolescents will reveal their own experiences with these emotions and thoughts.

We have been delivering the treatment in a group format (based on the UP-A manual's recommendations for a group format outlined in Chapter 23). This has been done for clinical and public health reasons. Since many of these youth report shame and stigma as a result of having SMI symptoms (e.g., Yang et al., 2015), we believed that providing the treatment in a group format would feel more supportive than individual treatment. Providing the treatment in a group format also increases access to care for adolescents, as more individuals can be seen in a session. Notably, a group format requires stricter adherence to the timeline of content delivery and a more fixed structure within each session. Otherwise, there is risk of not getting to each of the UP-A modules in the allotted treatment time. We decreased the number of sessions in the treatment from 16 to nine weekly outpatient sessions. Due to the relatively high rates of attrition in this population (Farris et al., 2020), it seemed prudent to reduce the total number of sessions in order to increase the rate of treatment completion. However, each session is extended from 50 minutes to 90 minutes, so the total time in treatment is virtually equivalent to the original UP-A. Of note, all of the core UP-A modules are still covered in our group format. We plan to extend the treatment to 12 sessions in future iterations to examine whether more time for acquisition and practice of therapeutic skills is acceptable and efficacious for participants.

Finally, we provide a parallel group treatment for parents of the adolescent participants, as is outlined for the Unified Protocol for Children (UP-C; Ehrenreich-May et al., 2017). At each session, the adolescents and parents convene in separate rooms for the first 75 minutes, and both groups are taught the same UP-A material. As is done in the UP-C, parents are also provided with information regarding (1) how they can improve their own emotional responses to their offspring's distress, (2) parenting behaviors that are effective versus ineffective for responding to their youth's distress, and (3) how they can best model and shape adaptive behaviors for their youth. In the final 15 minutes, the parents and adolescents are brought together into the same room, and each family individually meets in separate corners/areas of the room to make a game plan for when and where they will practice their skills. Once a game plan is decided, the family approaches a clinician to "check out" of the session, which involves sharing the plan for the next week, brainstorming any challenges/barriers, and attempting to overcome those challenges/barriers.

The purpose of including the parents in the treatment is multiple. First, the parents learn the treatment skills and are able to serve as a coach to their adolescents. Thus, parents can help to remind their adolescent to practice the skills and also facilitate the learning and practice of the skills. Second, a large proportion of the parents experience difficulties of their own with mood, anxiety, and SMI symptoms. Providing the treatment materials to the parents can be beneficial to the parents' mental health. Finally, we have found that including the parents in the treatment further normalizes the adolescents' psychiatric symptoms and engagement with the therapeutic skills. Since parents are asked to engage in each aspect of the treatment, the adolescents may feel less stigmatized by coming into treatment. Another bonus for some families is the increased cohesion that is built as a result of practicing the skills together.

TREATMENT CONSIDERATIONS

Our group-based UP-A is "billed" as a first-line psychosocial treatment for adolescents with SMI symptoms. The intention of our modified version of the UP-A is to provide clients with an introductory overview of the CBT skills. Thus, we primarily seek participants who have had little to no CBT previously. While this is not an absolute rule, clients who have come to us seeking treatment who have already undergone extensive CBT typically already know the skills we are teaching the group and commonly require more intensive individual-based treatment.

At the end of treatment, we make recommendations for the clients' next steps. Participants who feel equipped to use the skills on their own and have made significant progress in their symptoms and functioning typically terminate treatment and may not receive ongoing care. Participants who took to the treatment but want to receive continued CBT guidance most commonly seek individual-based CBT following our group. For clients who were non-responders, we have most commonly recommended family-focused therapy (FFT) and/or dialectical behavior treatment (DBT) programs. FFT helps to increase psychoeducation about psychiatric symptoms and improve communication and problem solving within the family (Miklowitz, 2010). Family treatment can be especially valuable for high-conflict families and has an evidence base for improving SMI symptoms in adolescents at high risk for psychosis and bipolar disorder. DBT is a more intensive CBT that can be especially useful for individuals with significant mood lability and self-harming behaviors (Linehan et al., 2007). This model of step-based care is similar to other clinical treatment programs (e.g., EPICENTER) that seek to provide initial low-intensity care followed by progressively higher-intensity and more disorder-specific treatment as the risk for SMI increases (Breitborde et al., 2020).

There have been a few requests from families to participate in another round of the group treatment. Although this is not absolutely prohibited, it is most commonly not recommended, as these participants have already learned the skills that will be presented. Thus, they will not be learning anything new when rejoining the group. However, in certain unusual circumstances in which participants had to drop out of treatment early or were otherwise not able to attend at least half of the sessions, we have allowed them to rejoin a later group.

Although we consider this treatment to be a first-line psychosocial treatment for adolescents with SMI symptoms, this treatment is most commonly done as an adjunct to pharmacotherapy. In fact, the vast majority of the participants have been prescribed psychiatric medication. However, this is not a requirement of our treatment. There have been situations in which we have recommended a medication consultation to families, but we leave medication decisions to families and their medical providers.

SUMMARY OF THE RESEARCH

Further rationale for the treatment and the details of preliminary findings from our first cohort who participated in the group treatment are reported elsewhere (Weintraub et al., 2020c). Since publishing this first report, we have held an additional three groups. In total, 14 youth–parent dyads have completed the treatment (out of 24 treatment initiators). These youth and their parents rated high levels of satisfaction ($M = 8.2$, $SD = 1.6$) and low levels of burden ($M = 2.0$, $SD = 2.1$) for the treatment on a 10-point Likert scale. When comparing pre- to post-treatment data of youth and parent reports, we found evidence of improvements in psychiatric symptoms, global functioning, and emotional regulation. Interestingly, homework compliance of skill practice (measured at each session) was associated with reductions in psychiatric symptoms and improved psychosocial functioning. These findings seem to suggest that the more the participants practiced their treatment skills, the better they got.

Unfortunately, compliance with the prescribed treatment skills is uniformly low across cognitive behavioral therapies (~50%; Gaynor et al., 2006), and the same was true in across our groups. Homework compliance in our first groups was about 47.1% (M weeks compliant = 3.8 out of 9 weeks, SD = 2.0). Since CBT's success hinges upon practice of treatment skills, we have become interested in methods to increase clients' motivation to practice the skills. In fact, our team at UCLA has begun developing a mobile app to facilitate the treatment. The app contains overviews of the session-by-session content, interactive skill practice, and symptom monitoring capabilities. It also has certain features to "gamify" the app, including rewards and levels participants can achieve, and notifications that remind participants to engage with the app and the treatment. While it remains unclear whether this strategy will be effective in increasing skill practice or treatment outcomes, we are excited to be putting these questions to the empirical test.

CASE EXAMPLE: JAMES

James is a 16-year-old male who met criteria for the attenuated psychosis syndrome due to unusual thoughts and suspiciousness that had worsened over the previous year. Specifically, he had thoughts that other people might be able to read his mind and that they may intend to harm him. His suspiciousness overlapped closely with his social anxiety disorder, in which he was consistently worried about what other people thought of him and was fearful to engage with peers. He also met criteria for major depressive disorder, current, single episode, which began at the start of his current school year. As a result of these symptoms, especially the social anxiety and suspiciousness, he withdrew from his regular public high school and began a homeschooling program. At the point of our intake assessment for the group treatment, he reported that he typically avoided leaving his house for fear he would have a social encounter. He also reported no friendships, although he indicated feeling close to his mother and older brother. His close relationship with his family proved to be a significant source of support and motivation for James throughout the treatment.

At the outset of treatment, he reported his goals were to feel less worried about other people's thoughts and intentions and to feel less depressed. James mentioned feeling significant guilt for his symptoms and expressed a motivation to feel better so that he would no longer be an emotional burden on his mother. James was quite shy and would be slow to warm up in each session. However, he was always compliant with the treatment team and would answer any questions that were asked of him. By the end of most sessions, he was fairly actively participating and would occasionally volunteer his opinion or answer questions.

The treatment starts with education around emotions and their function. This discussion appeared useful to James as it helped him put labels onto his feelings and helped him convey his feelings to his family. He also benefited from hearing about others' experiences in the early part of the treatment as he began to hear that others have had similar difficulties with anxiety and suspiciousness. Collectively, this module helped James feel more open to sharing his experiences with his family, which served as cathartic relief to him and allowed his family to better help James work through his difficulties throughout the treatment.

As the group progressed, James showed particular interest in the thinking strategies. He became very skilled at identifying his own thinking traps (and those of others), which were commonly "jumping to conclusions" and "catastrophizing." James mentioned that just by becoming aware of his thinking traps, he was able to calm himself down a little bit and begin to think more flexibly about the situation. While he was able to do the detective thinking and come up with alternative thoughts, James mentioned that it was the mindfulness section that was most helpful for him. He reported it was difficult to convince himself of alternative thoughts when he felt anxious or suspicious. However, he said that becoming more aware and accepting the thoughts as "just thoughts" (as opposed to trying to change them) helped him the most.

Of all of the modules, the behavioral module was where James's most visible improvements were made. With his goal of working through his anxiety and suspiciousness, we worked as a group to put together an emotion ladder that would facilitate this goal. He started by going for walks around the block at home with his mother a couple of times per week. He then started going for walks alone, and then going running alone. In parallel to his exercise regimen, he started going with his mother to small, relatively uncrowded stores during off-hours (early in the morning). By the end of the treatment, he began riding on the bus and, finally, went to a restaurant with his family for his birthday. While he reported that each of these steps was not easy, he was glad he did them and felt proud for pushing himself to do the exposures. Importantly, the cognitive module served as an important foundation for James as he began the behavioral strategies. He reported using those skills throughout his behavioral exercises as coping techniques.

By the end of the treatment, James's functioning was significantly improved, as he was slowly starting to reintegrate himself back into the community as well as exercise. He also reported improvements in his mood and anxiety. Although his unusual thought content and suspiciousness were still present, he indicated that he was better able to manage them. By the end of the treatment he said, "Just because I have a thought doesn't mean I need to believe it." Seemingly, the power of his prodromal thoughts was diminished even though they were still present.

TROUBLESHOOTING DIFFICULTIES

Treating youth at risk for SMI in a group setting presents some unique challenges. One is the initial reluctance of adolescents to share their SMI experiences, most notably unusual thought content, perceptual abnormalities, and grandiosity. It is important to note, however, that the adolescents do not need to share or discuss their SMI experiences with the group. Treatment can be successfully administered by the clinician and received by the adolescents without knowing their specific SMI experiences. However, sharing these experiences can facilitate the delivery of some of the skills (e.g., identifying thinking traps) and increase the cohesion of the group. To that end, a couple of strategies have proven helpful. First, it is recommended that the clinician present SMI experiences as relatively common among adolescents when going through treatment exercises (e.g., "Getting to Know Your Emotions") and use examples of SMI symptoms/ experiences throughout the treatment exercises. For example, when presenting common thinking traps, the clinician can share an example of a person who feels that other people might have negative intentions toward him or her and have the group identify what thinking trap(s) that thought might fall into. Second, it is recommended that the clinician ask the group whether anyone has ever felt much more irritable or elated for multiple days in a row, for example, or whether anyone feels suspicious of others at times. Again, these kinds of questions can fit in seamlessly with the "Getting to Know Your Emotions" exercise.

Another difficulty is getting the group members to reliably practice treatment skills and bring in their completed practice assignments. To help increase the likelihood of skill practice, we have the parents and teens, together, commit to a day and time that they will practice the skill. Further, we have the parents and teens work together to practice the skills. What that means is that both the parents and teens are asked to do the assignments. If the practice assignment is identifying and logging thinking traps, then both the parents and the teens write down thoughts and thinking traps that they encountered throughout their day. This helps to reduce the stigma of the treatment for the teens as well as promote the completion of the task. Additionally, we spend time in the beginning of each session (~15 to 20 minutes) to go through a homework review, where we ask each participant to raise their hand and share if they attempted to practice their skills that week. In line with behavioral reinforcement, this provides praise and attention for the teens who attempted skills.

A difficulty that commonly emerges in group treatments is balancing the needs of the individuals with the goal of getting the group through the treatment protocol. We have a few systems in place to ensure personalized attention for group members. First, we cap the groups at 12 participants, although a size of around six participants seems best for allowing each participant to share and receive individualized feedback. As we go through each session, we integrate games that help participants practice the skills and also allow the group leader to gauge their progress and provide individualized help and feedback. For example, after we introduce thinking traps, we have participants pick prewritten thoughts out of a hat and use their worksheet to figure out what thinking trap(s) that thought fits into. Or, for detective thinking, we assign group members a role—Unhelpful Thought Generator, Thinking Trap Identifier, Detective Question-er, and Alternative Thinker. They then go up to the whiteboard and, starting with the Unhelpful

Thought Generator (who comes up with any unhelpful/stressful thought he or she has experienced or can think of), they work through the detective thinking exercise. The participants are then randomly rotated through the various roles. Finally, as previously mentioned, we conduct homework review at the outset of each session and checkouts at the end of session so participants can get help solving any difficulties and making a game plan for the next week. While these strategies do not completely mitigate the need some adolescents will have for a more personalized, individual treatment, we believe that their implementation will help to guide the successful delivery of this treatment for many adolescents with early SMI symptoms.

Tip Sheet for Using the UP-A in Adolescents with Early SMI Symptoms

✓ **Why use UP-A for early SMI?**
- Emotional symptoms and disorders (i.e., depression and anxiety) are present in a large proportion of youth with SMI symptoms.
- UP-A can be used to address early SMI symptoms as well (i.e., unusual thought content and suspiciousness, grandiosity).
- UP-A can be a first-line psychosocial treatment. If the treatment skills gain traction in reducing symptoms and improving functioning, more intensive treatment may not be necessary. Otherwise, more intensive psychosocial and/or pharmacological therapy may be necessary.

✓ **How do I use UP-A for early SMI?**
- Start the treatment with "Weighing My Options" to help build motivation for engagement in treatment and to begin to formulate clear, measurable goals.
- Build awareness of emotions and a vocabulary to communicate about emotions and experiences with the "Emotion Identification Practice" and "Getting to Know Your Emotions." Follow these exercises with the skill of "I" statements to communicate emotions.
- Use the "Breaking Down My Emotions" worksheet and the "Tracking the Before, During, and After" form to help adolescents increase their understanding of the connection between their various experiences (thoughts, behaviors, and emotions). Present opposite action early and encourage behavioral activation/pleasurable activities within first few sessions.
- Incorporate SMI-specific examples when teaching the "Common Thinking Traps" and "Detective Thinking" (e.g., discuss suspiciousness in the context of jumping to conclusions).
- Develop interactive games for adolescents to practice the skills in session (e.g., draw a prewritten thought out of a hat and identify the thinking trap).
- Include deep breathing and/or a mindfulness breathing space in each session.
- Leverage detective thinking when having participants engage in opposite action.

✓ **What challenges might come up when using UP-A for SMI?**
- Adolescents may be reluctant to share their SMI symptoms/ experiences. Do your best to normalize SMI experiences, include examples of such experiences in your discussion, and be willing to ask adolescents if they have experienced them.
- Engagement with the treatment and progress throughout treatment will vary among adolescents in the group. Be sure to balance personalized attention (e.g., helping to solve an individual's difficulty with skill practice) with also making sure you complete the agenda for the session.

✓ **When is UP-A not appropriate for adolescents with SMI?**

- For adolescents with active suicidal thoughts or self-harm, a more intensive treatment option (e.g., dialectical behavior therapy) may be more appropriate.
- For those experiencing active psychotic or manic symptoms that would interfere with their ability to engage with the treatment or integrate with a group of peers, a more intensive treatment (most likely pharmacological treatment) and stabilization of symptoms would be needed prior to participation in treatment.

REFERENCES

Addington, J., Piskulic, D., Liu, L., Lockwood, J., Cadenhead, K. S., Cannon, T. D., Cornblatt, B. A., McGlashan, T. H., Perkins, D. O., Seidman, L. J., Tsuang, M. T., Walker, E. F., Bearden, C. E., Mathalon, D. H., & Woods, S. W. (2017). Comorbid diagnoses for youth at clinical high risk of psychosis. *Schizophrenia Research, 190*, 90–95.

American Psychiatric Association. (2013). *Diagnostic and statistical manual of mental disorders* (5th ed.). American Psychiatric Publishing.

Axelson, D., Goldstein, B., Goldstein, T., Monk, K., Yu, H., Hickey, M. B., Sakolsky, D., Diler, R., Hafeman, D., Merranko, J., Iyengar, S., Brent, D., Kupfer, D., & Birmaher, B. (2015). Diagnostic precursors to bipolar disorder in offspring of parents with bipolar disorder: A longitudinal study. *American Journal of Psychiatry, 172*(7), 638–646.

Beck, A. T., & Haigh, E. A. (2014). Advances in cognitive theory and therapy: The generic cognitive model. *Annual Review of Clinical Psychology, 10*, 1–24.

Birmaher, B., Axelson, D., Goldstein, B., Strober, M., Gill, M. K., Hunt, J., Houck, P., Ha., W., Iyengar, S., Kim, E., Yen, S., Hower, H., Esposito-Smythers, C., Goldstein, T., Ryan, N., & Keller, M. (2009). Four-year longitudinal course of children and adolescents with bipolar spectrum disorders: The Course and Outcome of Bipolar Youth (COBY) study. *American Journal of Psychiatry, 166*(7), 795–804.

Birmaher, B., Gill, M. K., Axelson, D. A., Goldstein, B. I., Goldstein, T. R., Yu, H., Liao, F., Iyengar, S., Diler, R. S., Strober, M., Hower, H., Yen, S., Hunt, J., Merranko, J. A., Ryan, N. D., & Keller, M. B. (2014). Longitudinal trajectories and associated baseline predictors in youths with bipolar spectrum disorders. *American Journal of Psychiatry, 171*(9), 990–999.

Breitborde, N. J., Guirgis, H., Stearns, W., Carpenter, K. M., Lteif, G., Pine, J. G., Storey, N., Wastler, H., & Moe, A. M. (2020). The Ohio State University Early Psychosis Intervention Center (EPICENTER) step-based care programme for individuals at clinical high risk for psychosis: study protocol for an observational study. *BMJ Open, 10*(1), e34031.

Brown, T. A., & Barlow, D. H. (2009). A proposal for a dimensional classification system based on the shared features of the DSM-IV anxiety and mood disorders: Implications for assessment and treatment. *Psychological Assessment, 21*(3), 256.

Duffy, A., Horrocks, J., Doucette, S., Keown-Stoneman, C., McCloskey, S., & Grof, P. (2013). Childhood anxiety: An early predictor of mood disorders in offspring of bipolar parents. *Journal of Affective Disorders, 150*(2), 363–369.

Ehrenreich-May, J., Kennedy, S. M., Sherman, J. A., Bilek, E. L., Buzzella, B. A., Bennett, S. M., & Barlow, D. H. (2017). *Unified protocols for transdiagnostic treatment of emotional disorders in children and adolescents: Therapist guide.* Oxford University Press.

Farris, M. S., Devoe, D. J., & Addington, J. (2020). Attrition rates in trials for adolescents and young adults at clinical high-risk for psychosis: A systematic review and meta-analysis. *Early Intervention in Psychiatry, 14*(5), 515–527.

Fusar-Poli, P., Bonoldi, I., Yung, A. R., Borgwardt, S., Kempton, M. J., Valmaggia, L., Barale, F., Caverzasi, E., & McGuire, P. (2012). Predicting psychosis: Meta-analysis of transition outcomes in individuals at high clinical risk. *Archives of General Psychiatry, 69*(3), 220–229.

Gaynor, S. T., Lawrence, P. S., & Nelson-Gray, R. O. (2006). Measuring homework compliance in cognitive-behavioral therapy for adolescent depression: Review, preliminary findings, and implications for theory and practice. *Behavior Modification*, *30*(5), 647–672.

Green, M. J., Cahill, C. M., & Malhi, G. S. (2007). The cognitive and neurophysiological basis of emotion dysregulation in bipolar disorder. *Journal of Affective Disorders*, *103*(1–3), 29–42.

Howes, O. D., & Murray, R. M. (2014). Schizophrenia: An integrated sociodevelopmental-cognitive model. *Lancet*, *383*(9929), 1677–1687.

Humphreys, K. (2017). A review of the impact of exclusion criteria on the generalizability of schizophrenia treatment research. *Clinical Schizophrenia & Related Psychoses*, *11*(1), 49–57.

Hutton, P., & Taylor, P. J. (2014). Cognitive behavioural therapy for psychosis prevention: A systematic review and meta-analysis. *Psychological Medicine*, *44*(3), 449–468.

Kessler, R. C., Chiu, W. T., Demler, O., & Walters, E. E. (2005a). Prevalence, severity, and comorbidity of 12-month DSM-IV disorders in the National Comorbidity Survey Replication. *Archives of General Psychiatry*, *62*(6), 617–627.

Kessler, R. C., Demler, O., Frank, R. G., Olfson, M., Pincus, H. A., Walters, E. E., Wang, P., Wells, K. B., & Zaslavsky, A. M. (2005b). Prevalence and treatment of mental disorders, 1990 to 2003. *New England Journal of Medicine*, *352*(24), 2515–2523.

Linehan, M. M., Bohus, M., & Lynch, T. R. (2007). Dialectical behavior therapy for pervasive emotion dysregulation: Theoretical and practical underpinnings. In Gross, James J. (Ed.), *Handbook of Emotion Regulation* (pp. 581–605). New York, US: Guilford Press.

McGlashan, T., Miller, T., Woods, S., Rosen, J., Hoffman, R., & Davidson, L. (2001). *Structured Interview for Prodromal Syndromes (SIPS)*. Yale University.

McGorry, P., & Nelson, B. (2016). Why we need a transdiagnostic staging approach to emerging psychopathology, early diagnosis, and treatment. *JAMA Psychiatry*, *73*(3), 191–192.

Miklowitz, D. J. (2010). *Bipolar disorder: A family-focused treatment approach*. Guilford Press.

Shaw, J. A., Egeland, J. A., Endicott, J., Allen, C. R., & Hostetter, A. M. (2005). A 10-year prospective study of prodromal patterns for bipolar disorder among Amish youth. *Journal of the American Academy of Child & Adolescent Psychiatry*, *44*(11), 1104–1111.

Sloan, E., Hall, K., Moulding, R., Bryce, S., Mildred, H., & Staiger, P. K. (2017). Emotion regulation as a transdiagnostic treatment construct across anxiety, depression, substance, eating and borderline personality disorders: A systematic review. *Clinical Psychology Review*, *57*, 141–163.

Wang, P. S., Lane, M., Olfson, M., Pincus, H. A., Wells, K. B., & Kessler, R. C. (2005). Twelve-month use of mental health services in the United States: Results from the National Comorbidity Survey Replication. *Archives of General Psychiatry*, *62*(6), 629–640.

Weintraub, M. J., Schneck, C. D., Axelson, D. A., Birmaher, B., Kowatch, R. A., & Miklowitz, D. J. (2020a). Classifying mood symptom trajectories in adolescents with bipolar disorder. *Journal of the American Academy of Child & Adolescent Psychiatry*, *53*(3), 381–390.

Weintraub, M. J., Schneck, C. D., Walshaw, P. D., Chang, K., Singh, M., Axelson, D., Birmaher, B., & Miklowitz, D. J. (2020b). Characteristics of youth at high risk for bipolar disorder compared to youth with bipolar I or II disorder. *Journal of Psychiatric Research, 123*, 48–53.

Weintraub, M. J., Zinberg, J. L., Bearden, C. E., & Miklowitz, D. J. (2020c). Applying a transdiagnostic unified treatment to adolescents at high risk for serious mental illness: Rationale and preliminary findings. *Cognitive and Behavioral Practice, 27*(2), 202–214.

West, A., Weinstein, S., & Pavuluri, M. N. (2017). Child-and Family-Focused Cognitive-Behavioral Therapy (CFF-CBT) for pediatric bipolar disorder. *Journal of the American Academy of Child & Adolescent Psychiatry, 56*(10), S348–S349.

Woods, S. W., Addington, J., Cadenhead, K. S., Cannon, T. D., Cornblatt, B. A., Heinssen, R., Perkins, D. O., Seidman, L. J., Tsuang, M. T., Walker, E. F., & McGlashan, T. H. (2009). Validity of the prodromal risk syndrome for first psychosis: Findings from the North American Prodrome Longitudinal Study. *Schizophrenia Bulletin, 35*(5), 894–908.

Yang, L. H., Link, B. G., Ben-David, S., Gill, K. E., Girgis, R. R., Brucato, G., Wonpat-Borja, A. J., & Corcoran, C. M. (2015). Stigma related to labels and symptoms in individuals at clinical high-risk for psychosis. *Schizophrenia Research, 168*(1), 9–15.

7

Substance Use Disorders

**FAITH SUMMERSETT WILLIAMS, REBECCA E. FORD-PAZ, AND
JASON WASHBURN ■**

Approximately half of all mental disorders that people experience over their life-time begin in adolescence (Kessler et al., 2007). In particular, the use of substances, including alcohol, marijuana, tobacco, illicit drugs, and prescription drugs, typically begins in adolescence. Earlier onset of substance use is associated with greater likelihood of developing a substance use disorder (Swendsen et al., 2012). Adolescents are more vulnerable than older adults to the addictive properties of nicotine, alcohol, marijuana, and other drugs, as their brains are still developing (Squeglia & Gray, 2016). When substance use disorders (SUDs) occur in adolescence, they affect key developmental milestones and often interfere with normal brain maturation (Squeglia & Gray, 2016).

The fifth edition of the *Diagnostic and Statistical Manual of Mental Disorders* (American Psychiatric Association, 2013) recognizes SUDs resulting from the use of 10 separate classes of drugs: alcohol, caffeine, cannabis, hallucinogens, inhalants, opioids, sedatives/ hypnotics/anxiolytics, stimulants, tobacco, and other or unknown substances. SUDs consist of cognitive, behavioral, and physiological symptoms resulting from the recurrent use of a substance despite functional and social impairment as a result of this use. Clinicians can specify the severity of an SUD, which is determined by the number of symptoms endorsed. The potentially lifelong consequences that result from an SUD diagnosis make addressing adolescent substance use a public health crisis.

The most commonly used substance among youth is marijuana. In 2011 approximately 66% of youth aged 12 to 17 received treatment for marijuana use compared to 43% for alcohol use, whereas it was the opposite for adults (Substance Abuse and Mental Health Services Administration, 2013). When teens drink alcohol, they are more likely than adults to binge drink (i.e., five or more drinks on a single occasion; Office of Applied Studies, 2008). Moreover, the use of electronic nicotine-delivery systems (ENDS), specifically electronic cigarettes (also known as e-cigarettes or vape devices), among young people aged 10 to 24 years has increased substantially in the past five years (Cullen et al., 2018). A recent study found that more than one-third of high school seniors in the United States report e-cigarette use in the past year (Gentzke et al., 2019). Available data suggest a strong association between ENDS and subsequent use of alcohol, marijuana, and other drugs (e.g., Curran et al., 2018).

The etiology of SUD in adolescence has been traced in part to untreated or undertreated internalizing disorders. Wolitzky-Taylor et al. (2012) found in a prospective study that baseline anxiety or depressive disorders predicted the onset of SUD. This is consistent with the "self-medication hypothesis" that those with depressive or anxiety disorders may seek to numb or alleviate their emotional distress through substance use (Khantzian, 1987). Adolescents who chronically use substances to alleviate psychological distress may underreport their substance use and be less likely to engage in treatment that seeks to eliminate or reduce it (Delaney-Black et al., 2010). Given that adolescents with substance use challenges often feel they do not need help, clinicians with expertise in integrated treatment for co-occurring psychopathology and substance use are highly recommended for this population (Brewer et al., 2017).

Despite the resistance to engaging in treatment for SUD, the available evidence suggests that youth in treatment have better outcomes than those not in treatment (Tanner-Smith et al., 2013). Interventions for adolescent substance use focus primarily on psychosocial interventions across individual, family, and group-based modalities. The intensity and duration of treatments vary from brief to extended multimodal interventions. The majority of efficacy and effectiveness research has evaluated office-based outpatient interventions, many of which were developmentally adapted from established adult treatments (Hogue et al., 2014). Adolescents with SUD differ from their adult counterparts in several ways and thus have different treatment needs (Winters et al., 1999). For instance, adolescents may be more susceptible to peer influences and may be more vulnerable to adverse effects from substances because of their biological, social, and cognitive stage in development (Bava & Tapert, 2010; Winters et al., 1999). Given these differences, interventions for adolescents that address multiple biopsychosocial targets are often more efficacious. Zero-tolerance approaches that promote abstinence from substances are ineffective among adolescents (Lynam et al., 1999). Abstinence-only approaches functionally deny services to those unwilling to completely eliminate use, which can be a barrier to treatment for adolescents who do not identify their substance use as problematic. As a result, harm-reduction approaches are more effective with adolescents because they acknowledge that experimentation is a normal part of adolescent development and offer strategies designed to reduce consequences of chronic use (Turner et al., 2014).

Several treatments have been shown to be efficacious for adolescents, including ecological family-based treatment, group cognitive-behavioral therapy (CBT), and individual CBT, with a modest amount of evidence supporting behavioral family therapy and motivational enhancement therapy (MET; Hogue et al., 2014). Substantial evidence supports combined treatment approaches that incorporate elements from the above-mentioned modalities to optimize treatment outcomes.

Among combined treatments, strong evidence supports combined MET and CBT, and combined MET, CBT, and behavioral family-based treatment (Hogue et al., 2014). Studies have found that outcomes are further enhanced by complementing the above-mentioned treatments with contingency management (CM). CM is a form of behavioral therapy based on operant conditioning principles. The purpose of CM in substance use treatment is to encourage pro-recovery behaviors through a system of tangible rewards for positive behaviors to reinforce those behaviors over time (Stanger et al., 2016). However, these treatments are limited in their focus on treating substance abuse in isolation, when comorbid psychopathology is more the rule than the exception. Research suggests that clients receiving integrated care for comorbid psychopathology and SUD fare better (Sterling & Weisner, 2005).

TRANSDIAGNOSTIC MODELS OF TREATMENT OF COMORBID SUD AND INTERNALIZING DISORDERS IN THE ADULT LITERATURE

Although evidence-based treatments for internalizing disorders and SUD have been dominated by single-disorder treatments (Farchione et al., 2018), there has been increasing interest in transdiagnostic interventions that target shared mechanisms across comorbid disorders (Kim & Hodgins, 2018). Such treatments might offer a more efficient, acceptable, and parsimonious model for clinicians to learn to treat substance use that co-occurs with other emotion-based disorders (Kim & Hodgins, 2018; Vujanovic et al., 2017). Transdiagnostic treatment approaches for SUD are based on the understanding that many forms of psychopathology, including SUD, are explained by transdiagnostic factors (Eaton et al., 2015). These factors are potentially optimal targets for therapeutic intervention efficiency (Barlow et al., 2011; Nathan & Gorman, 2002) as well as psychopharmacological interventions (Goldberg et al., 2011) and help explain why these treatments often alleviate symptoms of multiple disorders simultaneously. Additionally, transdiagnostic interventions could be more responsive and acceptable in real-world clinical settings where treatments for comorbid SUD and emotional disorders are in high demand (Ciraulo et al., 2013; Farchione et al., 2018).

Kim and Hodgins (2018) proposed a component model of addiction treatment that targets vulnerabilities across substance and behavioral addictions, including deficits in motivation to change, negative urgency (negative affect and impulsivity), deficits in self-control, expectancies (permissive and anticipatory beliefs) and motives (mood enhancement, social, coping), deficits in social support, and compulsive, maladaptive perseveration of addictive behaviors. Vujanovic et al. (2017) developed a theoretical framework targeting underlying cognitive-affective processes in both SUD and depression, focusing on negative affect, anhedonia, rumination, experiential avoidance, difficulties in emotion regulation, and distress tolerance. Similarly, other factors identified as underlying the prevalent comorbidity between internalizing disorders and SUD include neuroticism (Jackson & Sher, 2003) and emotion regulation difficulties (Kober, 2014).

Research on the effectiveness of transdiagnostic interventions for internalizing disorders and SUD remains in its infancy. Kushner et al.'s (2009) hybrid CBT protocol for anxiety and alcohol use disorder symptoms targets the links between anxiety and the motivation to drink, with evidence of improvement over a control group, as well as increased acceptability over single-disorder treatments. Baker et al. (2010) compared a single-disorder–focused CBT for depression or alcohol abuse with "integrated" CBT focused on both disorders, finding a greater reduction in drinking days and level of depression for integrated CBT compared to the single-disorder CBT intervention. Similarly, Riper et al.'s (2014) meta-analytic review of interventions combining CBT with motivational interviewing (MI) to treat comorbid alcohol use disorder and depression found small but clinically significant effect sizes in decreased depression symptoms and alcohol consumption at post-treatment.

The Unified Protocol for Transdiagnostic Treatment of Emotional Disorders (UP; Barlow et al., 2011) is a modular CBT intervention designed to address neuroticism, a core underlying factor of emotional disorders that helps to explain their frequent co-occurrence (including anxiety, depression, trauma- and stressor-related, obsessive-compulsive, and somatic disorders), as well as alcohol use disorders (Jackson & Sher, 2003). Neuroticism (defined as the tendency to experience frequent negative emotion and perceived uncontrollability or inability to cope; Barlow et al., 2014a) leads to strong negative reactions to emotions and maladaptive, avoidant coping (Barlow et al., 2014b). Although the UP was not originally designed as a standalone treatment for SUD, it overlaps with many of the treatment targets proposed in transdiagnostic treatment models for addictions and comorbid emotional disorders. For example, the UP modules focusing on motivational enhancement, emotional awareness, cognitive restructuring, reducing avoidant and maladaptive coping, and distress tolerance through situational emotion exposures reflect common elements between CBT for emotional disorders and SUD (Kim & Hodgins, 2018; Vujanovic et al., 2017). When substance use is the primary coping strategy to reduce negative mood states, it can be conceptualized as an avoidant coping behavior. Since the UP focuses on the development of more adaptive responses to emotions, individuals learn to tolerate intense emotions and somatic symptoms—such as withdrawal symptoms and cravings—in order to resist urges to use, while also adopting more goal-directed, adaptive behaviors (Farchione et al., 2018).

Similar to other transdiagnostic interventions, research on the efficacy of UP for comorbid SUD and emotional disorders is just beginning. In a study comparing four treatment conditions (UP + venlafaxine, progressive muscle relaxation + venlafaxine, UP + placebo, and progressive muscle relaxation + placebo [comparison group]) for adult clients with comorbid anxiety and alcohol use disorders, only the UP + placebo group demonstrated significantly decreased heavy drinking in contrast to the comparison group (Ciraulo et al., 2013). This study suggests that UP may have value in treating individuals with heavy drinking problems. Further research is needed to replicate these findings in adolescents and to examine the UP with other types of SUD.

ADAPTATION OF UP FOR SUD IN ADOLESCENTS

The United Protocol for Transdiagnostic Treatment for Emotional Disorders in Adolescents (UP-A) is likely to require adaptation when implemented for adolescents with comorbid emotional disorders and SUD. Before implementing the UP-A, it is important to assess for the severity and frequency of the adolescent's substance use. Screening measures, such as the Screening to Brief Intervention (S2BI; Levy et al., 2014) or the Brief Screener for Tobacco, Alcohol, and Other Drugs (BSTAD; Kelly et al., 2014), can be useful in identifying frequency of use and likelihood of a SUD in adolescents. In addition, brief assessments that evaluate the level of substance involvement and severity of substance-related problems are the CRAFFT (Car, Relax, Alone, Friends/Family, Forget, Trouble; Dhalla et al., 2011) and ASSIST (Alcohol, Smoking and Substance Involvement Screening Test; WHO ASSIST Working Group, 2002), which are validated among adolescents. When brief screening is highly suggestive of substance-related problems requiring intervention, a more thorough diagnostic interview is recommended to determine the presence/absence and severity of substance use as a disorder. Laboratory testing through human biological specimens such as blood, hair, salvia, or urine is often a useful, though imperfect, method used to complement self-report when evaluating adolescent substance use and tracking treatment progress.

Of note, adolescents with withdrawal symptoms may require a medically supervised detoxification program before engaging in the UP-A. Although the short length of stay of detoxification limits implementation of an inpatient version of the UP-A (Bentley et al., 2017), it is still possible to expose adolescents to some components of the UP-A. For example, detoxification programs could implement select modules or skills of the UP-A to increase motivation to change substance use behavior (Module 1), to provide psychoeducation on the emotional contributions to SUD (Module 2), or to teach some core UP-A skills (e.g., Notice It, Say Something About It, Experience It).

After assessment of SUD symptoms, and consistent with Module 1, the clinician is encouraged to use MI and other techniques to assess the adolescent's motivation to change substance use behaviors. Revisiting motivational enhancement techniques throughout treatment is common in the UP-A but may be especially important in its application to adolescent SUD to continually assess and maintain motivation, particularly in response to relapse.

When transitioning to Module 2, clinicians should work collaboratively with adolescents and their caregivers to identify the antecedent situations and individuals that increase the risk of engagement in substance use (i.e., the "before" of the "Tracking the Before, During, and After" form). Clinicians can help adolescents to develop strategies to minimize exposure to situations or individuals that increase the risk of substance use while they develop more adaptive responses to urges to use substances. During the early phases of treatment, it may be necessary to employ stimulus control and *temporarily* encourage avoidance of situations, people, and places that trigger the urge to use substances. Although experiential and emotional avoidance will be actively targeted in later modules of the UP-A, limiting an adolescent's exposure to situations and individuals that increase risk for engagement in substance use is necessary at the beginning of treatment (Ramo et al., 2012).

Psychoeducation can help adolescents and their caregivers better understand the impact of early substance use on biological, psychological, and social functioning, as well as the ways it negatively impacts current and future goals. Clinicians are encouraged to provide psychoeducation to adolescents and their families that conceptualizes substance abuse within the UP model. Specifically, clinicians should identify substance use as an emotional behavior and articulate the relationship between emotional distress and substance use as an emotional behavior. While depressed and anxious teens generally employ behavioral avoidance of emotionally taxing stimuli, those with comorbid SUD may be especially at risk for using substances to avoid emotional discomfort. Psychoeducation should emphasize that while substance use can offer a method for temporarily avoiding distressing and uncomfortable emotions, thoughts, and physiological responses, it can potentially increase mental health problems and emotional dysregulation, as well as risk for addiction, in the long term. Clinicians will likely need to integrate psychoeducation throughout treatment, highlighting the role of substance use as an emotional behavior while also emphasizing the physiological qualities of substances, such as cravings and withdrawal symptoms.

During Module 3, clinicians are encouraged to introduce the concept of values in addition to emotion-focused behavioral experiments and behavioral activation. Values are beliefs or principles that are important to an individual. Values are an important aspect of many psychotherapies, and clarification of the client's values has been found to be an effective element of treatments for adolescent substance use (Thurstone et al., 2017). Adolescents who use substances have often lost sight of their values because their behaviors are inconsistent with their core values. The clinician can demonstrate the connection between living in accordance with one's values and improved life satisfaction by encouraging the adolescent to practice behaviors that are more aligned with their values versus behaviors that are not (e.g., substance use or other emotional behaviors). By engaging in behavioral experiments and implementing "opposite actions" that align with their values, adolescents can experience firsthand how such behavioral choices have the capacity to impact mood.

In Module 4, clinicians are encouraged to revisit psychoeducation related to the somatic manifestations of distress (including triggers for substance use as well as cravings and withdrawal symptoms) and provide the rationale for sensational/interoceptive exposures using acceptance-based strategies. These strategies focus on helping adolescents to allow unwanted private experiences (general and withdrawal-specific thoughts, feelings, and urges) to come and go without struggling with them—without attempting to control or change them.

Module 5 incorporates cognitive techniques that have demonstrated efficacy in treating adolescent SUDs. Adaptations to this module should include psychoeducation on how to respond to frequently occurring negative thought patterns that trigger, exacerbate, and prolong substance use. Thoughts of inadequacy ("I'm not cut out for this") and inability to cope without the substance ("I need a drink to get through this") are likely to trigger use. Self-critical, black-and-white thinking about minor setbacks ("well, I've already had one broken promise to myself, I might as well keep going") often cause individuals to abandon attempts to reduce substance use. Additionally, state legalization of marijuana may fuel adolescents' beliefs about the benign nature of marijuana use and obscure its risks, increasing adolescent use. Adolescents would benefit from extra practice in implementing detective thinking skills to effectively challenge these thoughts and use problem-solving to generate alternative behavioral responses to break the connection between these thoughts and increased substance use.

Module 6 emphasizes mindfulness techniques and can be enhanced by incorporating acceptance strategies and explicitly exploring optimal times to employ these strategies as an opposite action to substance use. Acceptance-based strategies paired with mindfulness exercises that emphasize contact with the immediate environment can help adolescents learn to accept distressing thoughts, emotions, and physical sensations related to substance use. For example, exercises may be used to activate the senses through touch, sound, or taste to help the adolescent become aware of the here and now and to experience the moment with openness, interest, and receptiveness. It would be particularly beneficial to highlight that this is a technique to be used in moments of distress that would typically trigger substance use (e.g., anticipated stressful social situations, after experiencing disappointment or failure, during cravings). Building adolescents' capacity to observe their experience nonjudgmentally without impulsively engaging in the emotional behavior of numbing psychological distress with substances can allow the adolescent time and space to select a more values-driven behavior.

Module 7 may be adapted to include gradual cue exposure for SUD to expose youth to potentially triggering situations, places, and individuals to manage their cravings and reduce the potential for relapse. Conceptually, fear cues and cues for substance use are similar, and evidence for cue exposure therapy in the adult literature is encouraging (Byrne et al., 2019). In contrast, little is known about cue exposure for SUD in adolescents. Clinicians conducting cue exposures during Module 7 are encouraged to proceed with great care and introduce cue exposures only when adolescents have mastered emotion regulation skills and have had a period of successful relapse prevention. When engaging in cue exposures, it is important for clinicians to carefully monitor cravings and to develop and establish relapse prevention plans with adolescents and caregivers after a cue exposure session.

Implementation of the UP-A with adolescents with SUD may require a stronger family therapy component. Family-based treatments have been found to be particularly successful in treating adolescent substance use, in terms of improving both general positive parenting and parent management strategies specific to substance use, such as increased monitoring and limiting access to substances (Bo et al., 2018). Thus, clinicians are encouraged to expand the content of Module P by integrating a focus on family strengths and values, parent expectations and consequences, and family rituals, such as greetings, dinners, and games. Clinicians can work with caregivers and adolescents collaboratively to increase adolescent adherence to behavioral contingency programs or CM strategies designed specifically to reinforce pro-recovery behaviors and negative drug screens over time.

In Module 8 the clinician, adolescent, and caregivers prepare for treatment closure. Closure is an important part of the therapeutic process. Closure is important to review and reinforce the skills learned, plan for life with behaviors that are in accordance to healthy values, and create a relapse prevention plan that emphasizes substance use. Given the complexity of addressing SUD in adolescents, either as a primary condition or co-occurring with other emotional disorders, adolescents with SUD may require more time devoted to Module 8 to develop and monitor the implementation of relapse prevention plans.

CASE STUDY

The following case illustrates the elements of the UP-A that can be modified for successful treatment of SUD in adolescents. Brenda, a 16-year-old cisgender female whose parents moved from Puerto Rico to the mainland United States when she was an infant, was initially referred to treatment for depression. Treatment began with a standard implementation of the UP-A with a focus on depression and some co-occurring anxiety symptoms. Although Brenda was initially reserved, the clinician quickly developed rapport with her over the first two modules of the UP-A. At the start of Module 3, however, Brenda presented in a manner that strongly suggested that she was under the influence of marijuana. Although Brenda initially denied using marijuana, she eventually acknowledged having just "burnt one down" before her mother picked her up after school. Brenda initially dismissed any concerns about her substance use, stating that it was "under control." The clinician employed several strategies to address her resistance to acknowledging her substance use, such as amplified reflection, to eventually obtain Brenda's agreement to discuss her substance use in more detail. Using the BSTAD as a guide, the clinician identified that Brenda engaged in frequent use of alcohol (one or two times a week) and marijuana (one joint almost every day), although she denied symptoms of tolerance or withdrawal. The clinician also used the DSM-5 to assess for urges or cravings to use substances. Brenda reported a considerable level of craving for marijuana and a moderate level of craving for alcohol. The clinician then engaged Brenda in a discussion about disclosing her substance use to her parents, using the "Weighing My Options" worksheet from Module 1 of the UP-A. Although Brenda did not agree to disclose to her parents by the end of the session, she agreed to come back to therapy the next week to discuss it further.

Brenda arrived at the next session acknowledging that she was again under the influence of marijuana and immediately began crying. Brenda described substantial experiences of grief and guilt over the suicide of a friend with whom she had a "complex relationship." After some discussion, Brenda disclosed that she had been sexually involved with this friend and that the relationship was much more significant to her than she initially indicated. The clinician took this opportunity to integrate both her substance use and her grief into a revised clinical conceptualization. Specifically, the clinician helped Brenda to identify her emotional experience related to the loss of her friend as grief. Revisiting elements of Module 2, the clinician provided psychoeducation about grief, the function of grief, and the impact of grief on her symptoms of depression and her desire to use substances. Using the "Breaking Down My Emotions" worksheet, the clinician worked with Brenda to identify her grief-related thoughts, physical sensations, and behaviors. In particular, conceptualizing substance use as an emotion-driven behavior that served to avoid uncomfortable and distressing experiences of grief was critical for Brenda to acknowledge that her substance use may be related to her emotional experiences following the death of her close friend. At the close of this session, the clinician encouraged Brenda to complete the "Tracking the Before, During, and After" form when engaging in substance use.

At the subsequent session, the clinician was pleasantly surprised to see that Brenda had completed the form for two events over the past week. The clinician worked with Brenda to highlight how thoughts about her friend and distressing feelings associated with his loss preceded her urge to engage in substance use. The clinician took this opportunity to introduce the cycle of avoidance, highlighting how her substance use—a form of chemical avoidance—has increased, while her thoughts and feelings about the death of her close friend had not decreased. At the end of the session, the clinician revisited the "Weighing My Options" worksheet with Brenda, this time focusing on disclosing her substance use to her parents. With the new conceptualization of the interplay between her substance use and her distressing emotions, she agreed to disclose her substance use to her parents.

Although Brenda continued to report mild substance use on the BSTAD for several weeks—sometimes with her parents' awareness and other times without—she participated actively in treatment. The clinician returned to Module 3, integrating Brenda's substance use into the emotion-focused behavioral experiments. Before doing so, however, the clinician facilitated a discussion of values and completed a values card sort exercise with Brenda, who identified values of loyalty, respect, friendship, and self-control as her most important values. Identification of these values further strengthened her motivation to decrease her substance use. The values discussion led directly into completion of the "My Enjoyable Activities List," through which Brenda identified numerous prosocial activities with sober peers and adults, such as team sports. The clinician worked with Brenda and her parents to design behavioral experiments that increased the frequency of behaviors aligned with her value system using the "Weekly Activity Planner" and had Brenda track her emotional experiences using the "Emotion and Activity Diary."

The clinician also worked with Brenda's parents to increase monitoring and to modify situations that increased risk for substance use (e.g., staying up late on her phone). The increased structure was balanced with a discussion of the problems associated with common emotional parenting behaviors in response to substance use. The clinician used the "Double Before, During, and After" form to illustrate how their emotional responses to Brenda's substance use, such as overcontrol and criticism, were less effective than other responses. Instead, after re-emphasizing confidentiality, the clinician coached Brenda's parents in applying a harm reduction approach, helping them to understand that the goal is for Brenda to respond more effectively to her emotional experiences rather than to achieve immediate abstinence.

After addressing Brenda's unhelpful thinking patterns in Module 5, the clinician transitioned into Modules 6 and 7. The clinician engaged her in a discussion of how she could also use present-moment awareness techniques to slow down her emotional behavior of impulsively using substances to alleviate psychological distress. Brenda was then ready to start applying these skills to situations that historically triggered use (e.g., grief for her friend). Brenda was especially responsive to the "Emotion Story" exercise, focusing her written narrative on the loss of her close friend. By the time the clinician introduced situational emotion exposures in Module 7, such as driving by the house of her close friend who passed or reading his old text messages, Brenda was able to deal with the distress without engaging in emotion-driven behavior, including substance use. Shortly after implementation of these exposures, Brenda reported that she had stopped using substances. After reviewing her accomplishments along with her family, the clinician helped Brenda to develop a plan to prevent relapse into emotion-driven behavior and agreed to decrease her frequency of sessions to monthly check-ins that focused on psychoeducation, assessing relapse potential, and reinforcing alternatives to substance use for managing emotions. Although treatment extended for several months and was punctuated by a few relapses, Brenda eventually maintained her sobriety for an extended period of time and treatment was discontinued.

This brief case example illustrates the utility of the UP-A in addressing emotion-driven substance use, while also highlighting the barriers and facilitators to implementation with an adolescent client. Indeed, a particular challenge in conducting treatment of SUD in adolescents is when and how to involve parents in the treatment of substance use. Although in this case the client was motivated to disclose with the help of the tools provided in the UP-A and the skill of the clinician in MI, other adolescents may be unwilling to disclose, obliging the clinician to decide if it is necessary to break confidentiality. In some instances, it may not be worth damaging the therapeutic relationship by breaking confidentiality (e.g., experimentation with low risk of harm), while in other situations, it may be necessary to break confidentiality—against the wishes of the adolescent—to address concerns with safety (e.g., engaging in risky behaviors with substance use, combining lethal substances, or overdose). Clinicians implementing the UP-A with adolescents who use substances need to be prepared to address this issue,

particularly when motivational strategies are not successful in obtaining agreement from the client to disclose.

Clinicians should be aware of additional potential barriers in implementing
the UP-A with adolescents who use substances. In the case example, the parents
were engaged throughout the treatment, responded well to the concepts and skills
in Module P, and agreed to increase structure while not demanding abstinence.
Not all parents or caretakers will be available to engage in treatment, and not all
adolescents will have parents or caretakers. Further, some parents may have their
own difficulties with managing intense and distressing emotions that limit their
ability to reduce emotional parenting behaviors in favor of opposite parenting
behaviors. Finally, while some parents may reject a harm reduction model and in-
sist on immediate abstinence, other parents may struggle with their own substance
use or directly facilitate their adolescent's use of substances. In these situations,
clinicians should consider several alternatives, such as working more individually
with the adolescent, encouraging treatment for the parents or caretakers, or integrating more family-based components into the treatment.

Clinicians must also be careful about when—and if—to implement cue
exposures for substance use in Module 7. Although the case example illustrates
a successful implementation of exposures to situations that were triggers for
emotion-driven substance use, some adolescents may not have the stability or
skills to effectively respond to some cue exposures. Given how little we know about
cue exposure for substance use in adolescents, clinicians are encouraged to extend
the number of less-triggering graduated steps using the "My Emotion Ladder"
exercise to avoid a substance use response in an adolescent who is not sufficiently
prepared. In some situations, particularly when experiencing cravings, situational
avoidance of substance use cues may be necessary. Exposures that are "higher up
the ladder" should be reserved for when the adolescent has sufficient mastery of
the skills taught in the other modules of the UP-A, cravings are minimal, and the
adolescent has sufficient support and structure at home for monitoring and relapse prevention.

Tip Sheet for Using UP-A in Youth with SUDs

✓ **Why use UP-A for SUDs?**
- Substance abuse is often driven by the same transdiagnostic processes and emotional responses as other emotion-based disorders.
- The UP-A conceptualizes substance use as an avoidant behavior, helping adolescents and their families to understand the connection between the adolescent's emotional experiences and their substance use behavior.
- Substance use can be treated in the UP-A alongside other conditions, such as depression and anxiety.

✓ **How do I use UP-A for SUDs?**
- The tools and techniques in Module 1, such as the "Weighing My Options" worksheet, can be useful at the beginning of and throughout treatment in helping adolescents to develop and maintain motivation to address their substance use.
- The "Breaking Down My Emotions" worksheet and the "Tracking the Before, During, and After" form can be used to develop insight into the connection between distressing emotional experiences and engagement in substance use as an emotional behavior.
- The focus of Module 3 could be on the use of opposite action experiments in response to substance use cravings and the engagement in enjoyable and values-based activities that are incompatible with substance use.
- Increasing sensational awareness in Module 4 can be helpful in identifying somatic symptoms associated with cravings and withdrawal.
- Use the "Tracking the Before, During, and After" form to identify antecedents of substance use behavior, such as situational stressors and interpersonal difficulties, for which the "Getting Unstuck" worksheet can be used to aid in problem solving.
- Develop a safety plan to address the potential for overdosing or taking substances that may be tainted or spiked.

✓ **What challenges might come up when using UP-A for SUDs?**
- Substance use treatment will likely require more family therapy than is typical within the UP-A. Be prepared to work on increasing positive parenting to improve family functioning and relatedness more broadly, as well as substance-use–specific parenting strategies to increase monitoring and reduce access to substances.
- Some youth may not be ready for exposures related to substance use, while other youth may be ready but continue to avoid situational or interpersonal exposures. Help youth identify when they are ready to engage in cue exposures for substance use.
- Be prepared to continually revisit Module 1 throughout treatment.

✓ **When is UP-A not appropriate for youth with SUDs?**

- The UP-A may not be indicated for severe levels of SUD. Engage medical detoxification if the youth is demonstrating signs of tolerance or withdrawal symptoms. Higher levels of care (e.g., partial hospitalization, residential or inpatient) may also be necessary if the substance abuse worsens or become more risky, or if the youth experiences suicidal thoughts or behavior and persists with substance use.

REFERENCES

American Psychiatric Association. (2013). *Diagnostic and statistical manual of mental disorders* (5th ed.). American Psychiatric Publishing.

Baker, A. L., Kavanagh, D. J., Kay-Lambkin, F. J., Hunt, S. A., Lewin, T. J., Carr, V. J., & Connolly, J. (2010). Randomized controlled trial of cognitive-behavioural therapy for coexisting depression and alcohol problems: Short-term outcome. *Addiction, 105*, 87–99.

Barlow, D. H., Ellard, K. K., Sauer-Zavala, S., Bullis, J. R., & Carl, J. R. (2014a). The origins of neuroticism. *Perspectives on Psychological Practice, 9*(5), 481–496.

Barlow, D. H., Farchione, T. J., Fairholme, C. P., Ellard, K. K., Boissequ, C. L., Allen, L. B., & May, J. T. E. (2011). *Unified protocol for transdiagnostic treatment of emotional disorders: Therapist's guide.* Oxford University Press.

Barlow, D. H., Sauer-Zavala, S., Carl, J. R., Bullis, J. R., & Ellard, K. K. (2014b). The nature, assessment, and treatment of neuroticism: Back to the future? *Clinical Psychological Science, 2*, 344–365.

Bava, S., & Tapert, S. F. (2010). Adolescent brain development and the risk for alcohol and other drug problems. *Neuropsychology Review, 20*(4), 398–413.

Bentley, K. H., Sauer-Zavala, S., Cassiello-Robbins, C. F., Conklin, L. R., Vento, S., & Homer, D. (2017). Treating suicidal thoughts and behaviors within an emotional disorders framework: Acceptability and feasibility of the unified protocol in an in-patient setting. *Behavior Modification, 41*(4), 529–557.

Bo, A., Hai, A. H., & Jaccard, J. (2018). Parent-based interventions on adolescent alcohol use outcomes: A systematic review and meta-analysis. *Drug and Alcohol Dependence, 191*, 98–109.

Brewer, S., Godley, M. D., & Hulvershorn, L. A. (2017). Treating mental health and substance use disorders in adolescents: What is on the menu?. *Current Psychiatry Reports, 19*(1), 5.

Byrne, S. P., Haber, P., Baillie, A., Giannopolous, V., & Morley, K. (2019). Cue exposure therapy for alcohol use disorders: What can be learned from exposure therapy for anxiety disorders? *Substance Use & Misuse, 54*(12), 2053–2063.

Ciraulo, D. A., Barlow, D. H., Gulliver, S. B., Farchione, T., Morissette, S. B., Kamholz, B. W., Eisenmenger, K., Brown, B., Devine, E., Brown, T. A., & Knapp, C. M. (2013). The effects of venlafaxine and cognitive behavioral therapy alone and combined in the treatment of co-morbid alcohol use-anxiety disorders. *Behaviour Research and Therapy, 51*, 729–735.

Cullen, K. A., Ambrose, B. K., Gentzke, A. S., Apelberg, B. J., Jamal, A., & King, B. A. (2018). Notes from the field: Use of electronic cigarettes and any tobacco product among middle and high school students—United States, 2011–2018. *Morbidity and Mortality Weekly Report, 67*(45), 1276.

Curran, K. A., Burk, T., Pitt, P. D., & Middleman, A. B. (2018). Trends and substance use associations with e-cigarette use in US adolescents. *Clinical Pediatrics, 57*(10), 1191–1198.

Delaney-Black, V., Chiodo, L. M., Hannigan, J. H., Greenwald, M. K., Janisse, J., Patterson, G., Huestis, M. A., Ager, J., & Sokol, R. J. (2010). Just say "I don't": Lack of concordance between teen report and biological measures of drug use. *Pediatrics, 126*(5) 887–893. doi:10.1542/peds.2009-3059

Dhalla, S., D Zumbo, B., & Poole, G. (2011). A review of the psychometric properties of the CRAFFT instrument: 1999–2010. *Current Drug Abuse Reviews, 4*(1), 57–64.

Eaton, N. R., Rodríguez-Seijas, C. R., Carragher, N., & Krueger, R. F. (2015). Transdiagnostic factors of psychopathology and substance use disorders: A review. *Social Psychiatry and Psychiatric Epidemiology, 50,* 171–182.

Farchione, T. J., Goodness, T. M., & Williams, K. E. (2018). The Unified Protocol for comorbid alcohol use and anxiety disorders. In D. H. Barlow & T. Farchione (Eds.), *Applications of the unified protocol for transdiagnostic treatment of emotional disorders* (pp. 127–149). Oxford University Press.

Gentzke, A. S., Creamer, M., Cullen, K. A., Ambrose, B. K., Willis, G., Jamal, A., & King, B. A. (2019). Vital signs: Tobacco product use among middle and high school students—United States, 2011–2018. *Morbidity and Mortality Weekly Report, 68*(6), 157.

Goldberg, D., Simms, L. J., Gater, R., & Krueger, R. F. (2011). Integration of dimensional spectra for depression and anxiety into categorical diagnoses for general medical practice. In D. A. Regier, W. E. Narrow, E. A. Kuhl, & D. J. Kupfer (Eds.), *The conceptual evolution of DSM-5* (pp. 19–35). American Psychiatric Publishing.

Hogue, A., Henderson, C. E., Ozechowski, T. J., & Robbins, M. S. (2014). Evidence base on outpatient behavioral treatments for adolescent substance use: Updates and recommendations 2007–2013. *Journal of Clinical Child & Adolescent Psychology, 43*(5), 695–720.

Jackson, K. M., & Sher, K. J. (2003). Alcohol use disorders and psychological distress: A prospective state-trait analysis. *Journal of Abnormal Psychology, 112*(4), 599–613.

Kelly, S. M., Gryczynski, J., Mitchell, S. G., Kirk, A., O'Grady, K. E., & Schwartz, R. P. (2014). Validity of brief screening instrument for adolescent tobacco, alcohol, and drug use. *Pediatrics, 133*(5), 819–826.

Kessler, R. C., Amminger, G. P., Aguilar-Gaxiola, S., Alonso, J., Lee, S., & Ustun, T. B. (2007). Age of onset of mental disorders: A review of recent literature. *Current Opinion in Psychiatry, 20*(4), 359.

Khantzian, E. J. (1987). The self-medication hypothesis of addictive disorders: Focus on heroin and cocaine dependence. In D. F. Allen (Ed.), *The cocaine crisis* (pp. 65–74). Springer.

Kim, H. S., & Hodgins, D. C. (2018). Component model of addiction treatment: A pragmatic transdiagnostic treatment model of behavioral and substance addictions. *Frontiers in Psychiatry, 9,* 406.

Kober, H. (2014). Emotion regulation in substance use disorders. In J. Gross (Ed.), *Handbook of emotion regulation* (2nd ed., pp. 428–446). Guilford Press.

Kushner, M. G., Sletten, S., Donahue, P. T., Maurer, E., Schneider, A., Frye, B., & van Demark, J. (2009). Cognitive-behavioral therapy for panic disorder in patients being treated for alcohol dependence: Moderating effects of alcohol expectancies. *Addictive Behaviors, 34*(6–7), 554–560.

Levy, S., Weiss, R., Sherritt, L., Ziemnik, R., Spalding, A., Van Hook, S., & Shrier, L. A. (2014). An electronic screen for triaging adolescent substance use by risk levels. *JAMA Pediatrics, 168*(9), 822–828.

Lynam, D. R., Milich, R., Zimmerman, R., Novak, S. P., Logan, T. K., Martin, C., . . . Clayton, R. (1999). Project DARE: No effects at 10-year follow-up. *Journal of Consulting and Clinical Psychology, 67,* 590–593.

Nathan, P. E., & Gorman, J. M. (2002). *A guide to treatments that work* (3rd ed.). Oxford University Press.

Office of Applied Studies, Substance Abuse and Mental Health Services Administration. (2008, March 31). *Quantity and frequency of alcohol use among underage drinkers* (NSDUH Report). https://datafiles.samhsa.gov/

Ramo, D. E., Prince, M. A., Roesch, S. C., & Brown, S. A. (2012). Variation in substance use relapse episodes among adolescents: A longitudinal investigation. *Journal of Substance Abuse Treatment, 43*(1), 44–52.

Riper, H., Andersson, G., Hunter, S. B., de Wit, J., Berking, M., & Cuijpers, P. (2014). Treatment of comorbid alcohol use disorders and depression with cognitive-behavioural therapy and motivational interviewing: A meta-analysis. *Addiction, 109*, 394–406.

Squeglia, L. M., & Gray, K. M. (2016). Alcohol and drug use and the developing brain. *Current Psychiatry Reports, 18*(5), 46.

Stanger, C., Lansing, A. H., & Budney, A. J. (2016). Advances in research on contingency management for adolescent substance use. *Child and Adolescent Psychiatric Clinics, 25*(4), 645–659.

Sterling, S., & Weisner, C. (2005). Chemical dependency and psychiatric services for adolescents in private managed care: Implications for outcomes. *Alcoholism: Clinical and Experimental Research, 29*(5), 801–809.

Substance Abuse and Mental Health Services Administration. (2013). *Results from the 2012 National Survey on Drug Use and Health: Summary of national findings.* NSDUH Series H-46, HHS Publication No. (SMA) 13-4795.

Swendsen, J., Burstein, M., Case, B., Conway, K. P., Dierker, L., He, J., & Merikangas, K. R. (2012). Use and abuse of alcohol and illicit drugs in US adolescents: Results of the National Comorbidity Survey–Adolescent Supplement. *Archives of General Psychiatry, 69*(4), 390–398.

Tanner-Smith, E. E., Wilson, S. J., & Lipsey, M. W. (2013). The comparative effectiveness of outpatient treatment for adolescent substance abuse: A meta-analysis. *Journal of Substance Abuse Treatment, 44*(2), 145–158.

Thurstone, C., Hull, M., Timmerman, J., & Emrick, C. (2017). Development of a motivational interviewing/acceptance and commitment therapy model for adolescent substance use treatment. *Journal of Contextual Behavioral Science, 6*(4), 375–379.

Turner, R. A., Irwin Jr, C. E., & Millstein, S. G. (2014). Family structure, family processes, and experimenting with substances during adolescence. *Risks and Problem Behaviors in Adolescence, 1*(11), 229–247.

Vujanovic, A. A., Meyer, T. D., Heads, A. M., Stotts, A. L., Villareal, Y. R., & Schmitz, J. M. (2017). Cognitive-behavioral therapies for depression and substance use disorders: An overview of traditional, third-wave, and transdiagnostic approaches. *American Journal of Drug & Alcohol Abuse, 43*(4), 402–415.

WHO ASSIST Working Group. (2002). The Alcohol, Smoking and Substance Involvement Screening Test (ASSIST): Development, reliability and feasibility. *Addiction, 97*(9), 1183–1194.

Winters, K. C., Latimer, W. L., & Stinchfield, R. D. (1999). Adolescent treatment. In P. J. Ott, R. E. Tarter, & R. T. Ammerman (Eds.), *Sourcebook on substance abuse: Etiology, epidemiology, assessment, and treatment* (pp. 350–361). Allyn and Bacon.

Wolitzky-Taylor, K., Bobova, L., Zinbarg, R. E., Mineka, S., & Craske, M. G. (2012). Longitudinal investigation of the impact of anxiety and mood disorders in adolescence on subsequent substance use disorder onset and vice versa. *Addictive Behaviors, 37*(8), 982–985.

8

Avoidant/Restrictive Food Intake Disorder

KRISTINA DUNCOMBE LOWE AND SARAH ECKHARDT ■

POPULATION AND SETTING

With the publication of the fifth edition of the *Diagnostic and Statistical Manual of Mental Disorders* (DSM-5; American Psychiatric Association [APA], 2013), the conceptualization of eating disorders has continued to expand in an effort to better encapsulate the full range of symptoms in clients with disordered eating. Eating disorders, in general, are particularly harmful for youth because of the many negative effects, including malnutrition, growth retardation, loss of cognitive functioning, changes in emotional functioning, and even premature death (Campbell & Peebles, 2014; Franko et al., 2013; Herzog et al., 2000).

Each eating disorder diagnosis varies in weight presentation, eating behaviors, and course of treatment (Table 8.1). Several eating disorders are characterized by both body image concerns and restrictive eating patterns aimed at altering one's shape or weight (anorexia nervosa, bulimia nervosa), while others are described by their avoidant and restrictive eating behaviors without body image concerns (avoidant/restrictive food intake disorder [ARFID]). ARFID is characterized by avoidant or restrictive eating behavior that results in one or more of the following:

1. Significant weight loss (or failure to achieve expected growth),
2. Nutritional deficiency,
3. Dependence on oral nutritional supplements or enteral feeding, and/or
4. Significant interference with psychosocial functioning.

Clinical traits of the disorder include lack of interest in food, avoidance of food due to aversive sensory characteristics, and concern over negative outcomes of eating (e.g. vomiting, choking; APA, 2013). In addition to having several symptom

Table 8.1 EATING DISORDER DESCRIPTIONS

Eating Disorder	Weight Status	Eating Pattern	Body Image Concerns	Compensatory Behaviors
Anorexia nervosa	Underweight	Restrictive	Yes	May be present, but not diagnostically necessary
Bulimia nervosa	Typically normal weight	Restrictive and binging	Yes	Yes, part of diagnostic criteria
Avoidant/restrictive food intake disorder	Can present as underweight or normal weight	Restrictive and avoidant	No	No
Binge eating disorder	Typically overweight	Binging/loss of control	Yes	No

presentations, recent findings have indicated that symptom presentations often overlap and co-occur (Duncombe Lowe et al., 2019).

Diagnostic rates for clients with ARFID are still being determined, given that it was only added to the most recent edition of the DSM. However, while most eating disorders have higher prevalence rates among females, ARFID affects a greater number of males than does anorexia nervosa or bulimia nervosa, and it appears that ARFID clients are younger and have a longer duration of illness before diagnosis (Fisher et al., 2014).

Current front-line outpatient treatments for anorexia nervosa and bulimia nervosa include family-based treatment (FBT) and cognitive-behavioral therapy (CBT) (Fairburn et al., 2003; Le Grange & Lock, 2009; Lock & Le Grange, 2013). Additionally, the Unified Protocol for Transdiagnostic Treatment of Emotional Disorders (Barlow et al., 2017) was recently adapted by Thompson-Brenner et al. (2018) to address eating disorder symptoms and co-occurring psychopathology in clients treated at the residential level of care. It was generally considered potentially efficacious at ameliorating emotional disorders associated with eating disorders. Less is known about evidence-based treatments for the newer diagnosis of ARFID. Current work on the treatment of ARFID primarily focuses on single approaches aimed at treating specific clinical categories within ARFID (e.g., picky eating) or adapting existing eating disorder treatments in an attempt to fit the needs of children and adolescents with ARFID (Mammel & Ornstein, 2017). Since the most promising adaptations thus far appear to be treatments utilizing FBT and CBT principles (Fitzpatrick et al., 2015; Mammel & Ornstein, 2017), and because our treatment team has endeavored to adapt and tailor the Unified Protocols for Transdiagnostic Treatment of Emotional Disorders in Children and Adolescents (UP-C/A) for this newly identified client population, this chapter will focus specifically on the combined approach of FBT with the UP-C/A for the treatment of youth with ARFID.

Recent findings suggest that the negative consequences of ARFID can mirror the negative effects of anorexia nervosa, in that youth with ARFID can present with similar physical complications, including low weight, severe malnutrition, stunted growth, cardiac complications, delayed menstruation, and gastrointestinal difficulties (Fisher et al., 2014; Nicely et al., 2014; Strandjord et al., 2015). Children with ARFID also present to hospital emergency departments with major medical and physical complications at a similar rate to clients with anorexia nervosa (Fisher et al., 2014). Additional findings suggest ARFID clients are more likely to have a comorbid medical condition, which puts children with ARFID at significant risk for health complications when compared to other eating disorder clients (Fisher et al., 2014; Strandjord et al., 2015). Common psychological comorbidities of ARFID include generalized anxiety, obsessive-compulsive disorder, learning disorders, cognitive impairment, and neurodevelopmental disorders, such as autism spectrum disorder and attention-deficit/hyperactivity disorder (Nicely et al., 2014). Recent research suggests that comorbid disorders among youth with ARFID may be related to shared transdiagnostic constructs of their specific clinical presentation (Kambanis et al., 2019). For example, Kambanis et al. (2019) found that youth with ARFID who presented with sensory sensitivity characteristics had greater odds of having a comorbid neurodevelopmental, anxiety, obsessive-compulsive, depressive, bipolar-related, trauma-related, or disruptive/conduct disorder when compared to youth with ARFID displaying other clinical characteristics (e.g., fear of aversive consequences, lack of interest in eating). Given that ARFID is a relatively new diagnosis, more information on specific medical and psychological comorbidities, including how they impact treatment, is needed (Katzman et al., 2019). Additionally, because of the unique tendency for youth with ARFID to present with both medical and psychological symptoms, treatment should focus on addressing both aspects of the diagnosis by utilizing FBT to empower parents and increase weight to a healthy range, while frequently adding the UP-C/A to help clients address avoidant/restrictive behaviors, fears about trying new foods, and physical sensations associated with eating, as well as common comorbid emotional disorders, including anxiety and depressive disorders.

APPLYING A UP CASE CONCEPTUALIZATION TO ARFID

Several mechanisms addressed by the UP-C/A appear to be a good fit when conceptualizing change in clients with ARFID. Specifically, ARFID clients frequently exhibit high reactivity to trying many foods/eating, as well as strong physical sensations (e.g., fullness, stomach pain/discomfort) that affect their ability to eat. The UP-C/A is also helpful in addressing distress tolerance, as clients frequently have difficulty tolerating exposures to new foods or the strong emotions/sensation that can come up when challenging their eating. Clients with ARFID may also make attempts to avoid, suppress, or escape negative emotions; the UP-C/A can help decrease this avoidance by teaching clients to approach food with consistency and evaluate the before, during, and after of their emotional response. The UP-C/A provides clients with the ability to learn ways to become more aware of uncomfortable physical sensations associated with eating and to tolerate those feelings through sensational exposures.

ADAPTATIONS TO UP-C/A FOR ARFID

What makes treating eating disorders unique is the necessity for the intervention to address the weight challenges as well as the psychological and behavioral aspects associated with the eating disorder. In order to treat the physical, psychological, and behavioral concerns commonly seen in ARFID, the UP-C/A can be used in conjunction with several sessions of FBT. FBT is generally used for the first two or more sessions to assess the impairment around eating, to separate the illness from the child, to provide psychoeducation about regular eating and the effects of malnutrition/low weight, to empower parents to feed their child effectively, and to unite families in helping their child recover from their eating disorder. For some families, the UP-C/A may then be added between Sessions 2 and 4, while other families may not be ready until a later session (Figure 8.1). The total number of sessions for the combined FBT and UP treatment typically lasts between 12 and 20 sessions. Once the UP-C/A is added to treatment, the session consists of time spent checking in on both FBT principles, including solving problems with refeeding or regular eating if necessary, and the UP-C/A sessions/modules.

Specific adaptations to the UP-C/A consist of psychoeducation on the effects of being malnourished/underweight, the benefits of regular eating, and the importance of helping the youth recover from the eating disorder. Education is also provided on the importance of altering the child's current behaviors that are causing psychosocial impairment. For example, a therapist may discuss the child's fears of eating and how they have impacted the family's life, given that the child can no longer eat at friends' houses or restaurants. Providing hope and education on how to normalize the child's eating is included throughout sessions to guide how behavioral experiments are conducted. For example, behavioral experiments may include eating what a friend eats at a play date or having the family eat at a restaurant that the child does not typically eat at. Some families will have difficulty knowing what goals to set to normalize their child's eating because much of their life has been adapted to make accommodations for their child's eating issues. In these cases, psychoeducation on developmentally appropriate norms around eating is important.

Another key adaptation to the UP-C/A for ARFID is the focus of at least one Top Problem on the client's specific eating problem. For example, a client with extreme selective eating symptoms may endorse a Top Problem of "Only able to eat certain foods/lack of variety with eating." The SMART goal for this problem may then be to add three new foods to the child's diet over the next three months.

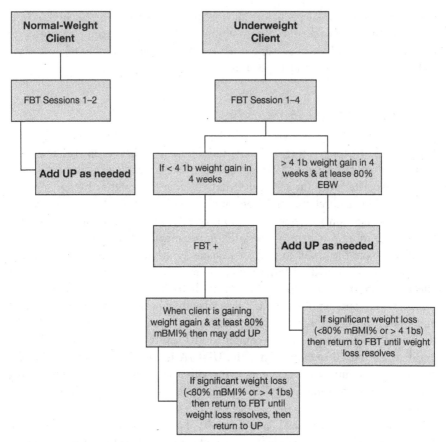

Figure 8.1. Treatment Decision Tree

Another way that treatment for youth with ARFID may differ from other disorders is that once a client has begun food exposures, it is recommended that the client engage in daily food exposures at home with parental support from that point on. This is recommended because high levels of fears around food often impair regular day-to-day eating for youth with ARFID; as such, helping them habituate to appropriate eating habits and foods requires a focused and consistent effort. Exposures are usually recommended as part of the therapy sessions going forward as well, in order to model for youth and parents how to conduct appropriate exposures and to encourage families to learn the skills to approach new/more challenging foods on their own. Repeated exposures to the same foods are also recommended because most youth with ARFID will not habituate to foods after one sitting. Since most youth will not "like" the food after only a few tries, education on how to tolerate eating the food is provided and clients are praised for being able to tolerate foods. This concept is further explored in cognitive flexibility sessions/modules, where clients are encouraged to be flexible about the outcomes of eating particular foods.

Food exposures should be unique to the client and their specific aversions. It is helpful to make a hierarchy based on the client's specific difficulties, with particular focus on helping the client tolerate their concern, whether it be taste, texture, or something else. Research has shown an increase in child acceptance of previously disliked foods after repeated exposures to the same food (Fildes et al., 2014). Studies have shown parents should present new or disliked foods between eight and 15 times in order to increase a child's acceptance (Carruth et al., 2004). A hierarchy for a youth with sensory aversions to taste and texture should start small, building the child's confidence in their ability to tolerate disliked foods. For example, a youth with a very limited diet may start their food hierarchy by choosing three foods they would like to add to their diet or selecting three foods that are similar to foods they already eat. Once those foods are chosen, each food has its own hierarchy as the youth repeatedly tries to work up the food exposure ladder until they can tolerate eating a whole portion size. The youth may work for several weeks on adding one food, and this is appropriate as long as they are working up their food exposure ladder at each presentation. To decrease burnout of a particular food, it may be helpful to rotate food exposures so that the repeated exposure of the same food occurs every two or three days. This may mean the youth works on two or three foods concurrently, depending on the youth, their parents, and the overall feasibility of different daily exposures. Some families may prefer to work on one food at a time, which can also be appropriate. While many youth are able to improve eating through repeated exposures aimed at their particular concern (e.g., taste, texture), it is important to note that youth with high levels of disgust may struggle to habituate to foods due to a heightened sensitivity to taste (Harris et al., 2019).

Another common challenge for some youth with ARFID is an overarching difficulty tolerating foods unless they are presented in a very specific way. This may mean that the foods have to be a particular brand or that the texture (perfect amount of crisp or softness), presentation (has to look the same), and/or temperature (hot or cold) have to be "just right." For youth with these types of sensory aversions, it is helpful to focus on tolerating foods in a variety of ways, including building the hierarchy around eating a specific food with more flexibility. For example, a child who likes chicken nuggets but will only eat them if they are a specific brand, shape, and temperature (warm) may start exposures by trying their preferred chicken nuggets at different temperatures, and then working up to new shapes and brands until they are able to tolerate several different variations.

It is critical to allocate specific time to prepare parents to provide appropriate support and guidance to their child during exposures. For various reasons, exposures can be stressful and/or difficult for both parents and youth, which in turn can increase both parties' avoidance of them. Providing appropriate education, training, and support to parents early on is vital to the success of exposures at home. Parent education and training should focus on helping parents respond with both neutrality and warmth to their child's fears/discomfort around food, praising and rewarding their child for participation and showing effort during the exposure, and being firm with expectations that the child will participate in the exposure process and continually push their level of comfort. Parents should encourage youth to go at least one step beyond their current comfort level with the food. For example, a parent whose child is comfortable smelling a particular food but is highly averse to putting the food in their mouth may encourage their child to work through their fears by moving up the exposure ladder (e.g., licking the food). Parents may have difficulty finding an appropriate level of guidance, as some will want to push too much and others will want to push too little. Assessing the specific family's needs in this area will help you appropriately guide and support parents in finding the right amount of support. Helping parents respond to exposures with neutrality and warmth is very important, as many parents are reactive to their child's responses around food and/or eating. Instead of having parents react as they normally would to a child in distress, the goal is to encourage them to respond with neutral kindness but not accommodation if their child becomes distressed or defiant or demonstrates physical distress (e.g., vomiting, gagging) during exposures. It is important to help the parents know that their child is distressed because of the anxiety or difficulty around eating and that their discomfort and distress can reduce with exposure and encouragement. For example, if a child is distressed about trying a food and begins to gag, it can be helpful to model for the parents and child that it is normal to become physically distressed when they are trying hard things and validate that the child is doing something challenging, while also encouraging them to continue with the exposure. It may also be appropriate to provide reassurance to the parents that their child's physical response is not a true anxiety alarm warning them of danger but rather a trained response that can be retrained to more adaptive eating habits. Modeling all of these characteristics will be helpful in the beginning of treatment.

Once you have engaged the parent in leading exposures, it may be helpful to prepare them before the home exposures (without the child present) and to debrief with them after, as some youth will demonstrate high reactivity to the exposures and parents may need support and reassurance that they handled it appropriately.

Most of the published worksheets from the UP-C/A (Ehrenreich-May et al., 2017) are compatible when working with youth with ARFID, as you can generally choose a problem to focus on and set up treatment around the specific eating difficulty. For example, sensational exposures are very helpful to start the process of helping youth recognize that their physical sensations around eating are natural, normal, and not harmful. Starting with the non-food–related exercises in the UP-C/A is helpful, but it may also be crucial for the child to start doing sensational exposures around food. For example, sensational exposures aimed at ARFID clients might include having clients drink fluids until their stomach feels full to practice coping with feelings of fullness/fears of something bad happening if their stomach is full or having clients hold food in the back of their mouth to cope with sensations they associate with choking or the need to vomit.

In addition to the UP-C/A worksheets, a Food Exposure Ladder is created (Figure 8.2). The Food Exposure Ladder is used to help youth during exposures, as they are encouraged to start at the bottom and work their way up the ladder for

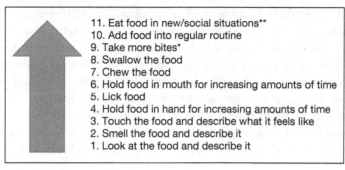

11. Eat food in new/social situations**
10. Add food into regular routine
9. Take more bites*
8. Swallow the food
7. Chew the food
6. Hold food in mouth for increasing amounts of time
5. Lick food
4. Hold food in hand for increasing amounts of time
3. Touch the food and describe what it feels like
2. Smell the food and describe it
1. Look at the food and describe it

Figure 8.2. Food Exposure Ladder
mBMI%, percent median body mass index; % of expected body weight (EBW).
*This step can also include taking bigger bites, as most youth with ARFID start with
very small bites and need encouragement to take regular-sized bites. **This step is
where youth are encouraged to try eating these newly added/or re-added foods in more
situations, such as at school, a friend's house, or a restaurant.

each exposure until that food is regularly eaten (or eaten in a specific place regularly). After a child becomes comfortable with exposures, it is common for them to skip ahead and start on a harder step of the food ladder. They may revert to the first step for more challenging exposures.

Therapists work with the child/adolescent and parent to encourage them go one step beyond what ARFID "wants them to." However, it is also important to end sessions on a positive note and try to make each exposure successful in one way or another. For example, if a child was unable to work past a certain point with the food and was highly distressed, the therapist should praise the youth for what they did well with and point out how they are building up their tolerance to sit with difficult emotions or make their own decisions instead of "allowing ARFID to decide." One exercise that can be particularly helpful during exposures is asking the youth to use mindfulness or present-moment awareness skills to nonjudgmentally approach the food. For example, you may guide the youth to notice, say something, and experience the food without judgment during the exposure, praising them for tolerating the experience.

APPROPRIATENESS OF UP-C/A AS INTEGRATED FIRST-LINE INTERVENTION, ADJUNCTIVE INTERVENTION, OR ALTERNATIVE INTERVENTION

The UP-C/A may serve as an integrated first-line treatment with FBT in most cases for youth with ARFID, as FBT focuses on restoring weight/health, and the UP-C/A addresses the emotional and behavioral issues associated with disordered eating and comorbid emotional disorders. In cases where clients are of normal weight and are already eating, the UP-C/A is an appropriate integrated front-line treatment for youth with ARFID. In cases where the client is underweight or not eating regularly, it can be used as an adjunctive intervention to FBT. The UP (Barlow et al., 2017) has already been used as an alternative intervention for eating disorder clients diagnosed with a variety of eating disorders (e.g., anorexia nervosa, bulimia nervosa, binge eating disorder), with pilot data supporting that the implementation may benefit transdiagnostic outcomes for clients enrolled in residential treatment (Thompson-Brenner et al., 2018). The UP-C/A may also serve as an adjunctive treatment with FBT in most cases for youth with ARFID, as FBT focuses on restoring weight/health, and the UP-C/A addresses the emotional and behavioral issues associated with disordered eating and comorbid emotional disorders.

For clients with eating disorders who present as underweight, whether it be the result of recent weight loss or more chronic weight concerns, the UP-C/A may or may not be appropriate, depending on the client's current medical needs and symptoms of food avoidance (see Figure 8.1). As such, FBT focused on empowering parents to help their child gain/restore weight is the recommended first-line treatment for youth with eating disorders who are underweight or malnourished. FBT is also the recommended first-line treatment for clients with eating disorders who are developmentally unable to engage in cognitive treatment and/or oppositional to weight restoration or change.

BRIEF SUMMARY OF RELEVANT RESEARCH DATA

There is a scarcity of published treatment research on efficacious treatments for ARFID due to its very recent addition to the DSM-5. Data exist for the effectiveness of treatments aimed at more general eating and feeding disturbances, but the efficacy of these treatments for ARFID is still unknown. Research on the treatment of ARFID is currently limited to case studies/series, retrospective chart reviews, and three small randomized controlled trials in a very specialized population of children (Lock et al., 2019; Sharp et al., 2016, 2017). Most recently, Thomas et al. (2020) completed an open trial for ARFID clients aged 10 to 17 years, which was the first study to evaluate the feasibility, acceptability, and proof-of-concept for their manualized CBT approach. However, these preliminary intervention approaches have yet to be rigorously evaluated (Mammel & Ornstein, 2017), highlighting the growing need to establish a first-line treatment for this diagnosis.

While some research has attempted to address the heterogeneous symptoms of ARFID, a treatment model that also incorporates the full range of commonly comorbid disorders (e.g., depression, anxiety) into one cohesive, flexible, and adaptable approach is needed. There is a critical need for an evidence-based treatment (EBT) that can address both the behavioral aspects of ARFID and its concomitant emotional disorders. Without an EBT for ARFID, even clinicians with a high degree of expertise in treating eating disorders may be left to adapt or create other untested treatment models for this disorder (Thomas et al., 2018). Moreover, clinicians with less expertise in eating disorders may feel unprepared to treat ARFID altogether. A recent meta-analysis suggested that out of 600 ARFID clients, providers included nutritional therapists, pediatricians, psychologists, and speech and occupational therapists (Sharp et al., 2017). Because ARFID clients are often seen by several providers across many settings, it is vital for an EBT for ARFID to be developed that can be easily disseminated to different specialties/ settings in order to increase access to evidence-based care among ARFID clients. Not only do these findings suggest that it is imperative to establish an efficacious EBT approach for ARFID, but they also, more specifically, suggest the need for an EBT that takes into account the wide variations (e.g., selective eaters, fears of vomiting/choking) in clinical presentation, as well as the comorbid emotional disorders frequently seen in children and adolescents with ARFID, that can be generalized and disseminated to clinicians with child/adolescent/family backgrounds in order to enhance optimal, evidence-based care for these clients.

Research suggests that a course of treatment for ARFID that addresses both malnutrition and underlying anxiety and mood disorders that lead to food aversions (Bryant-Waugh, 2013; Kenney & Walsh, 2013) may be the most effective treatment for this complex disorder. Together, FBT and the UP-C/A target these heterogeneous symptoms and therefore address major clinical characteristics that make treatment of ARFID challenging. That is, FBT can be utilized to stabilize weight and regular eating while the UP-C/A can be utilized to treat comorbid emotional disorders and avoidance symptoms.

A recent case study by our treatment team (Eckhardt et al., 2019) presented evidence on the use of FBT, combined with the UP-C, for a client diagnosed with ARFID, separation anxiety disorder, and a specific phobia of choking. At the end of treatment, improvements were seen in the client's weight and willingness to eat a full range of foods. Decreases in anxiety regarding eating/choking, fears of food being contaminated with gluten, and fears of eating while being away from parents were also observed. These findings highlighted initial promising results from this combined treatment approach for ARFID. Our team also continues to participate in an open case series of ARFID clients in two different treatment settings (Calgary, Canada, and Melbourne, Australia) and is working toward publishing preliminary data for clients treated in our clinic utilizing strictly FBT versus FBT combined with the UP-C/A.

CASE EXAMPLE

"Amanda" is a 10-year-old girl presenting with weight loss and food avoidance. She has a history of worrying about her performance, safety of herself and family, and social situations. Her parents report that she has always been a somewhat picky eater but that she had no difficulties eating regular meals with her family and keeping up with appropriate weight gains until six months ago. At that time, Amanda took a large bite of chicken and thought she was choking. Following that incident, she started avoiding solid foods and eating much less, leading to a rapid 10-pound weight loss. She also started avoiding meals with her family, would not eat in front of friends, and would not eat anywhere but at home with at least one parent present. Though her parents tried to help her get back to her normal diet and routine, Amanda was resistant and would rather skip meals than eat "unsafe" foods in different places or with other people.

A thorough assessment, including a semistructured clinical interview with Amanda and her parents, as well as self and parent report on the Multidimensional Anxiety Scale for Children, 2nd Edition (MASC-2; March, 2012) and the Children's Depression Inventory 2 (CDI-2; Kovacs, 2011). yielded diagnoses of ARFID and generalized anxiety disorder.

Prior to Session 1, Amanda was medically cleared for outpatient care by her primary care physician. A dietitian calculated her percent median body mass index using her growth charts and found that Amanda had typically been tracking along the 40th percentile for her age, gender, height, and weight. While Amanda had only lost 10 pounds since the onset of her eating difficulties, she needed to gain at least 15 pounds in order to return to the 40th percentile (because she had also grown). Because Amanda had a significant amount of weight to gain, treatment initially utilized FBT to empower her parents to help Amanda eat enough food to gain one pound per week (until reaching her weight goal), using her currently preferred foods. After four weeks, and four pounds of weight gain, the UP-C was then added into her treatment.

Amanda and her parents agreed on the following Top Problems and goals:

1. Problem: Limited variety in diet because of fears/many lost foods that are no longer acceptable
   Goal: Add back in 10 previously eaten meals within the next six months.
2. Problem: Not eating in certain situations because of fears
   Goal: Become able to eat without parents in room, in the car, at school, and with friends within the next six months.
3. Problem: High anxiety in other areas (safety, performance, social situations)
   Goal: Learn five new coping skills in the next six months to use to cope with anxiety.

As is common in this population, subsequent sessions focused on both continuing to increase weight and addressing Amanda's UP-C Top Problems. After Sessions 2 through 5 were presented, exposures were incorporated into treatment. Exposure work was moved up in treatment due to the high level of impairment in eating that was making regular eating and gaining weight challenging. To help Amanda identify her emotional behaviors for each problem area, she completed the "Emotional Behavior" form. For example, one of her situations was "Not eating solid foods," which she identified led to the emotional behavior of "avoidance and angry outbursts." She rated these emotional responses as a 7 out of 8 on the emotion scale. Amanda was able to use the coping skills she developed from the UP-C to add several solid foods back into her regular diet within two months. The participation in daily food exposures was vital to her success, as she learned to tolerate different tastes, textures, and physical sensations associated with food. This was important because it not only helped Amanda face her fears about choking on solid foods but also allowed for the addition of more variety into her diet that made it easier for her to restore the lost weight.

Before trying food exposures, Amanda and her therapist made an individualized ladder of how to try new foods. This ladder was different than the fear ladder as it was based specifically on learning to try new or previously accepted foods (see Figure 8.2). Amanda was able to work up her ladder for trying new foods and was able to start eating solid foods in the home setting. Once she was able to do this, exposures focused on helping her eat solid foods in new situations and without her parents present. These exposures were challenging for Amanda, and it was helpful to use detective thinking. Consider the following dialog:

> *Amanda:* I can't eat chicken nuggets for lunch at school because I might choke.
> *Therapist:* That sounds like a really scary thought. I wonder if it might be a thinking trap. Maybe we could use your detective thinking skills to evaluate whether that is the most realistic interpretation of the situation?
> *Amanda:* I can try, but I really don't want to eat chicken nuggets for lunch.
> *Therapist:* I like that you're willing to try. Let's start by seeing if you are falling into any thinking traps. What do you think?
> *Amanda:* I think I might be "Jumping to Conclusions" because I don't actually know that I will choke if I eat chicken nuggets for lunch.
> *Therapist:* That's a good guess. How about we start looking for evidence as to whether or not you would choke during lunch if you had chicken nuggets?
> *Amanda:* Well . . . some evidence might be that I've had chicken nuggets before and I haven't choked.
> *Therapist:* That's a great piece of evidence. What other evidence do you see?
> *Amanda:* My friends eat chicken nuggets for lunch.
> *Therapist:* And what happens to your friends when they eat chicken nuggets for lunch?
> *Amanda:* Nothing. They like eating chicken nuggets.
> *Therapist:* OK, so you've had chicken nuggets for lunch before and you did not choke, and your friends eat chicken nuggets for lunch and they don't choke. Given the evidence you just pointed out, do you think your thought about choking on chicken nuggets is the most realistic thought?
> *Amanda:* No, I guess not.
> *Therapist:* So if that's not the most likely thing to happen, maybe we can use your problem-solving steps to find a more realistic thought?

TROUBLESHOOTING AND BARRIERS

There are some particular challenges associated with use of the UP-C/A in clients with eating disorders. In particular, given the medical risks that can be associated with youth with ARFID, treating this population typically requires specialists who can address the client's low weight and malnutrition, in addition to their emotionally driven avoidant behaviors. Collaboration with the client's medical team to understand their medical stability, as well as set appropriate goals for weight gain, is vital. The problem with helping clients who are underweight (either chronically or acutely) to approach broader eating goals, without addressing their underlying malnutrition, is that they will continue to be at risk for medical difficulties, lack of growth, and so forth. FBT is therefore a very important adjunctive treatment in order to help clients gain weight and establish appropriate regular eating habits first. Working closely with the client's medical team to ensure appropriate weight gain and renourishment is established is vital before the UP-C/A can be added. Because this is a population that is typically seen by specialty clinics, it can make seeking treatment difficult, as the hours and access to the clinic may be more limited than in other behavioral health settings.

COMMON CONCERNS WITH THIS POPULATION

- Clients who have recently lost a significant amount of weight may need medical stabilization through the hospital before being cleared for outpatient treatment. **Suggestion:** Have clients seek care and ensure medical stability prior to starting outpatient treatment.
- Severely underweight clients may require extensive refeeding (and weight gain) before they are cognitively ready to participate in the UP-C/A. **Suggestion:** Give clients time to recover medically from the effects of being underweight before having them participate in cognitive treatment. Some clients may need to gain weight and eat regularly for several months before they have the capacity to engage in the UP-C/A.
- Since motivation and health status for youth with ARFID may vary, strong parental involvement throughout all the stages of the UP-C/A is encouraged. This is particularly true during exposures around food, which are a critical part of the treatment in this population. **Suggestion:** Have discussions with all caregivers about the need for consistency in essential areas of treatment (e.g., gaining weight, use of UP-C/A strategies, daily exposures). Some caregivers choose to work together to create a consistent routine. For clients living in multiple households, both caregivers may require the youth to complete a food exposure daily, but the foods the child eats and the rewards the youth can earn at each house may be different. Additionally, some families may choose to complete exposures and use UP-C/A strategies at only one parent's home.
- Sometimes youth present with chronic eating problems (and even chronically low weight/medical problems) but they and their families have adapted to living with ARFID and are not motivated to make changes. **Suggestion:** Approaching this at two points during treatment

is important in helping families move through their ambivalence. The first point is during the first few sessions of FBT, where you provide education about the effects of being underweight/malnourished and the importance of helping their child improve their health. Using the "intense scene" common to FBT is vital in helping clients and parents feel more motivated to face the issues around eating and health that they have been accommodating for a long time. The second point is during the first module of the UP-C/A, where families set goals and then evaluate the pros and cons of making changes versus not making changes. Motivational interviewing techniques are employed to move families toward change talk. Note: After going through these steps, some families will decide that it is not worth the challenges to make the changes they have come to treatment to address. Suggesting that the family take some time and consider participating in treatment at a later point may be appropriate; however, if the child is underweight or malnourished, it is important to continue recommending the family face the challenges of weight gain at this time.

- Teenage clients who have chronic eating problems, including clients who have had longstanding issues with selective eating due to disliking the taste and textures of foods, can have problems establishing motivation to add more foods in. Even though clients might acknowledge that being able to eat a larger variety of foods would help them physically and psychosocially, they may have a hard time believing that anything will change for them. **Suggestion:** UP-A Module 1 is especially important for these clients; it may take several sessions in order to establish motivation to make changes to their eating or even provide hope that such a feat is possible. The "Tracking the Before, During, and After" form are also very valuable for helping youth realize the patterns they are stuck in compared to what their life could be like if they did things in a different way.

Tip Sheet for Using UP-C/A in Youth with ARFID

✓ **Why use UP-C and UP-A for ARFID?**
  - UP-C and UP-A can address negative emotions and distressing physical sensations associated with both ARFID and comorbid disorders that may contribute to eating difficulties.
  - UP-C and UP-A can address avoidant behaviors seen around eating, as well as other unhelpful coping strategies to avoid experiencing strong emotions. It can help clients learn to tolerate their emotions when eating new foods or in new places with new people.
  - Common problems seen in ARFID populations, including difficulties coping with physical sensations associated with strong emotions, can be addressed in UP-A Module 4 or UP-C Session 4 through sensational exposures.

✓ **How do I use UP-C and UP-A for ARFID?**
  - Use the "Breaking Down My Emotions" worksheet and the "Tracking the Before, During, and After" form to help youth develop insight into their unhelpful patterns around eating.
  - Use opposite action, detective thinking, and experiencing body clues early and often!
  - Some youth with ARFID are generally avoidant of all strong emotions. Using the modules/sessions on emotional awareness and how to cope with emotions is helpful in building up their tolerance for emotions in general and emotional reactions to eating.
  - For youth with very avoidant or restrictive eating habits, adding situational exposures into each session fairly early in treatment is helpful. We recommend adding them in after UP-A Modules1 through 5 or UP-C Sessions 1 through 5 have been covered so that clients have the skill base to tolerate difficult emotions associated with exposures.

✓ **What challenges might come up when using UP-C and UP-A for ARFID?**
  - Some youth struggle to act opposite because they have experienced ARFID their whole lives and may take time to buy into the idea that their symptoms can improve. Make sure that the activities you choose for initial opposite action experiments are small and achievable. You may need help from caregivers to encourage the client to engage.
  - Exposures may be especially challenging for youth with ARFID and may require extra support from parents to make engaging in difficult food challenges positive. For example, using a reward system may be helpful because youth with ARFID may not always have internal motivation to make changes.

✓ **When is UP-C or UP-A most appropriate for youth with ARFID?**
  - The youth has worries and fears that interfere with age-appropriate eating.
  - The youth has specific rules or rituals around eating that are difficult to change.
  - The youth has a comorbid emotional disorder that needs to be treated in conjunction with the eating disorder.

✓ **When is UP-C or UP-A not appropriate for youth with ARFID?**
  - The youth has severe medical complications or psychological comorbidities that require a higher level of care.
  - The youth lacks motivation to engage in their own treatment. In these cases, FBT is more appropriate.

REFERENCES

American Psychiatric Association. (2013). *Diagnostic and statistical manual of mental disorders* (5th ed.). American Psychiatric Publishing.

Barlow, D. H., Farchione, T. J., Sauer-Zavala, S., Latin, H. M., Ellard, K. K., Bullis, J. R., Bentely, K. H., Boettcher, H. T., & Cassiello-Robbins, C. (2017). *Unified protocol for transdiagnostic treatment of emotional disorders: Therapist guide*. Oxford University Press.

Bryant-Waugh, R. (2013). Avoidant restrictive food intake disorder: An illustrative case example. *International Journal of Eating Disorders, 46*, 420–423.

Campbell, K., & Peebles, R. (2014). Eating disorders in children and adolescents: State of the art review. *Pediatrics, 134(3)*, 582–592.

Carruth, B., Ziegler, P., Gordon, A., & Barr, S. (2004). Prevalence of picky eaters among infants and toddlers and their caregivers' decisions about offering a new food. *Journal of the American Dietetic Association, 104*, 57–64.

Duncombe Lowe, K., Barnes, T. L., Martell, C., Keery, H., Eckhardt, S., Peterson, C. B., Lesser, J., & Le Grange, D. (2019). Youth with avoidant/restrictive food intake disorder: Examining differences by age, weight status, and symptom duration. *Nutrients, 11(8)*, 1955.

Eckhardt, S., Martell, C., Lowe, K. D., Le Grange, D., & Ehrenreich-May, J. (2019). An ARFID case report combining family-based treatment with the unified protocol for transdiagnostic treatment of emotional disorders in children. *Journal of Eating Disorders, 7(1)*, 34.

Ehrenreich-May, J., Kennedy, S. M., Sherman, J. A., Bennett, S. M., & Barlow, D. H. (2017). *Unified protocol for transdiagnostic treatment of emotional disorders in adolescents: Workbook*. Oxford University Press.

Ehrenreich-May, J., Kennedy, S. M., Sherman, J. A., Bilek, E. L., & Barlow, D. H. (2017). *Unified protocol for transdiagnostic treatment of emotional disorders in children: Workbook*. Oxford University Press.

Ehrenreich-May, J., Kennedy, S. M., Sherman, J. A., Bilek, E. L., Buzzella, B. A., Bennett, S. M., & Barlow, D. H. (2017). *Unified protocols for transdiagnostic treatment of emotional disorders in children and adolescents: Therapist guide*. Oxford University Press.

Fairburn, C. G., Cooper, Z., & Shafran, R. (2003). Cognitive behaviour therapy for eating disorders: A "transdiagnostic" theory and treatment. *Behaviour Research and Therapy, 41(5)*, 509–528.

Fildes, A., van Jaarsveld, C., Wardle, J., & Cooke, L. (2014). Parent-administered exposure to increase children's vegetable acceptance: A randomized controlled trial. *Journal of the Academy of Nutrition and Dietetics, 114(6)*, 881–888.

Fisher, M. M., Rosen, D. S., Ornstein, R. M., Mammel, K. A., Katzman, D. K., Rome, E. S., Callahan, S. T., Malizio, J., Kearney, S., & Walsh, T. (2014). Characteristics of avoidant/restrictive food intake disorder in children and adolescents: A "new disorder" in DSM-5. *Journal of Adolescent Health, 55(1)*, 49–52.

Fitzpatrick, K. K., Forsberg, S. E., & Colborn, D. (2015). Family-based therapy for avoidant restrictive food intake disorder: Families facing food neophobias. In K. L. Loeb, D. Le Grange, & J. Lock (Eds.), *Family therapy for adolescent eating and weight disorders* (pp. 256–276). Routledge.

Franko, D. L., Keshaviah, A., Eddy, K. T., Krishna, M., Davis, M. C., Keel, P. K., & Herzog, D. B. (2013). A longitudinal investigation of mortality in anorexia nervosa and bulimia nervosa. *American Journal of Psychiatry, 170*(8), 917–925.

Harris, A. A., Romer, A. L., Hanna, E. K., Keeling, L. A., LaBar, K. S., Sinnott-Armstrong, W., Strauman, T. J., Wagner, H. R., Marcus, M. D., & Zucker, N. L. (2019). The central role of disgust in disorders of food avoidance. *International Journal of Eating Disorders, 52*(5), 543–553.

Herzog, D. B., Greenwood, D. N., Dorer, D. J., Flores, A. T., Ekeblad, E. R., Richards, A., Blais, M. A., & Keller, M. B. (2000). Mortality in eating disorders: A descriptive study. *International Journal of Eating Disorders, 28*(1), 20–26.

Kambanis, P. E., Kuhnle, M. C., Wons, O. B., Jo, J. H., Keshishian, A. C., Hauser, K., Becker, K. R., Franko, D. L., Misra, M., Micali, N., Lawson, E. A., Eddy, K. T., & Thomas, J. J. (2020). Prevalence and correlates of psychiatric comorbidities in children and adolescents with full and subthreshold avoidant/restrictive food intake disorder. *International Journal of Eating Disorders, 53*(2), 256–265.

Katzman, D., Norris, M., & Zucker, N. (2019). Avoidant restrictive food intake disorder. *Psychiatric Clinics of North America, 42*, 45–57.

Kenney, L., & Walsh, T. (2013). Avoidant/restrictive food intake disorder (ARFID): Defining ARFID. *Eating Disorders Review, 24*(3).

Kovacs, M. (2011). *Children's depression inventory 2 (CDI-2)*. Multi-Health Systems, Inc.

Le Grange, D., & Lock, J. (2009). *Treating bulimia in adolescents: A family-based approach*. Guilford Press.

Lock, J., & Le Grange, D. (2013). *Treatment manual for anorexia nervosa: A family-based approach*. Guilford Press.

Lock, J., Robinson, A., Sadeh-Sharvit, S., Rosania, K., Osipov, L., Kirz, N., Derenne, J., & Utzinger, L. (2019). Applying family-based treatment (FBT) to three clinical presentations of avoidant/restrictive food intake disorder: Similarities and differences from FBT for anorexia nervosa. *International Journal of Eating Disorders, 52*(4), 439–446.

Mammel, K. A., & Ornstein, R. M. (2017). Avoidant/restrictive food intake disorder: A new eating disorder diagnosis in the Diagnostic and Statistical Manual 5. *Current Opinion in Pediatrics, 29*, 407–413.

March, J. S. (2012). *Multidimensional anxiety scale for children, Second Edition (MASC-2)*. Multi-Health Systems, Inc.

Nicely, T. A., Lane-Loney, S., Masciulli, E., Hollenbeak, C. S., & Ornstein, R. M. (2014). Prevalence and characteristics of avoidant/restrictive food intake disorder in a cohort of young patients in day treatment for eating disorders. *Journal of Eating Disorders, 2*, 21.

Sharp, W. G., Allen, A. G., Stubbs, K. H., Criado, K. K., Sanders, R., McCracken, C. E., Parsons, R. G., Scahill, L. S., & Gourley, S. L. (2017). Successful pharmacotherapy for the treatment of severe feeding aversion with mechanistic insights from cross-species neuronal remodeling. *Translational Psychiatry, 7*(6), e1157.

Sharp, W. G., Stubbs, K. H., Adams, H., Wells, B. M., Lesack, R. S., Criado, K. K., Simon, E. L., McCracken, C. E., West, L. L., & Scahill, L. D. (2016). Intensive, manual-based intervention for pediatric feeding disorders: Results from a randomized pilot trial. *Journal of Pediatric Gastroenterology and Nutrition, 62*(4), 658–663.

Sharp, W. G., Volkert, V. M., Scahill, L., McCracken, C. E., & McElhanon, B. (2017). A systematic review and meta-analysis of intensive multidisciplinary intervention for pediatric feeding disorders: How standard is the standard of care? *Journal of Pediatrics, 181,* 116–124.

Strandjord, S. E., Sieke, E. H., Richmond, M., & Rome, E. S. (2015). Avoidant/restrictive food intake disorder: Illness and hospital course in patients hospitalized for nutritional insufficiency. *Journal of Adolescent Health, 57,* 673–678.

Thomas, J. J., Wons, O. B., & Eddy, K. T. (2018). Cognitive–behavioral treatment of avoidant/restrictive food intake disorder. *Current Opinion in Psychiatry, 31*(6), 425–430.

Thompson-Brenner, H., Boswell, J. F., Espel-Huynh, H., Brooks, G., & Lowe, M. R. (2018). Implementation of transdiagnostic treatment for emotional disorders in residential eating disorder programs: A preliminary pre-post evaluation. *Psychotherapy Research, 29*(8), 1045–1061.

9

Pediatric Illnesses and Pediatric Settings

RYAN R. LANDOLL, KADE B. THORNTON, AND
CORINNE A. ELMORE[1] ∎

Childhood is a crucial developmental period where mild psychological symptoms can present increased risk for disruptions in later functioning in adulthood. Therefore, targeting emotional concerns in youth by using prevention and intervention efforts is essential. Transdiagnostic treatments provide a flexible treatment option by addressing shared symptom components across diagnoses. They can be used with clients who present with comorbidities or subclinical symptoms or who do not fit into clear-cut diagnostic categories (Boisseau et al., 2010). The Unified Protocols for Transdiagnostic Treatment of Emotional Disorders (UP; Barlow et al., 2011) and versions for children and adolescents (UP-C/A; Ehrenreich-May et al., 2017) include core principles for treatment of emotional disorders. These treatments address shared components of emotional disorders by focusing on how clients experience, respond to, and regulate difficult emotions rather than on specific diagnoses. This chapter will review how the UP-C/A can be applied specifically in pediatric populations, focusing on both illnesses and settings.

A review of the literature on applications of the UP-C/A to comorbid mental illness and physical illnesses that commonly affect children shows that applications have primarily focused on correlates of anxiety and sympathetic arousal, including somatic complaints as well as more significant and chronic pain concerns. Biological sensitivity to stress, as described by Weersing et al. (2012), can lead to a heightened sensitivity to pain and emotional distress. Physical complaints

1. **Author's Note:** This chapter was authored in part by employees of the United States government. Any views expressed herein are those of the authors and do not necessarily represent the views of the United States government or the Department of Defense.

such as abdominal pain, headaches, muscle tension, and chest pain without medical cause are extremely common in childhood (Masia-Warner et al., 2009). Children who experience somatic complaints are at risk of reduced school attendance, poor academic functioning, and school refusal behaviors (Hughes et al., 2008). Further, somatic complaints in childhood can lead to chronic pain in adulthood (Gureje et al., 2001). Often these children will seek medical help without detection or treatment of their psychological symptoms. As emotional regulation difficulties often precede these somatic complaints, there is possibly shared risk for some medical conditions and internalizing disorders—and shared benefit in addressing pain and emotional distress via the UP-C/A (Kroenke & Swindle, 2000).

In addition to the literature on comorbid mental and physical illness, there has also been an increased focus in behavioral health care within integrated health care settings (Vogel et al., 2017). Thus, it will be important to understand how the UP-C/A may be adapted not only for comorbid health conditions but also in diverse health care settings. Despite the high prevalence rates of childhood emotional disorders (Mojtabai et al., 2016; Rapee et al., 2009), symptoms of anxiety and depression are frequently unrecognized or underdiagnosed, especially in primary care settings (Barbui & Tansella, 2006). Several factors contribute to these treatment rates, including lack of access to care, lack of detection, and lack of knowledge about appropriate treatment (Allen et al., 2020). Consequently, providing treatment solely in specialty behavioral health settings will not adequately meet the need. A current approach has been to offer these treatments where children already access other services.

PEDIATRIC HEALTH CONDITIONS

The estimated prevalence of children with a chronic physical health condition is nearly 25% (Cleave et al., 2010). The adverse effects of chronic physical conditions can be severely distressing for children. In addition to the distress of pain or discomfort, chronic medical conditions often lead to missed school, an inability to continue social or physical activities, and added family stress. To complicate matters further, behavioral health concerns disproportionately affect children with chronic health conditions. It has been estimated that nearly half of children with significant physical health problems suffer from comorbid psychiatric conditions (Canning et al., 1992), creating a significant barrier to the successful treatment of chronic physical health conditions among youth (Butler et al., 2018). Indeed, increased rates of behavioral problems, as well as symptoms of depression and anxiety, are commonly reported among children who suffer chronic physical illnesses such as asthma, diabetes, and chronic pain issues (Quach & Barnett, 2015).

In addition to reducing mental health symptoms, an increasing body of literature demonstrates that psychological treatments make a significant impact on improving treatment adherence and, in some cases, diminishing physical symptoms (Li et al., 2017; Yorke et al., 2007). Indeed, cognitive-behavioral approaches have been used to successfully treat chronic pain (headaches and abdominal pain) in children (Eccleston et al., 2014), reduce panic symptoms as well as physical symptoms of asthma (Deshmukh et al., 2007), and improve treatment adherence for children diagnosed with diabetes (Li et al., 2017). In addition to supplementing care for a variety of medical diagnoses, psychological interventions have also proven useful in ameliorating medically unexplained somatic symptoms (Reigada et al., 2008).

While the link between physical and mental health may be robust, significant barriers to effectively managing these comorbidities remain. First, despite the high co-occurrence of physical and mental health concerns among children, symptoms of anxiety and depression are not often recognized by primary care providers (Barbui & Tansella, 2006), nor are parents as comfortable discussing mental health concerns with their child's pediatrician (Briggs-Gowan et al., 2000). This is compounded by a lack of training in mental health competencies in medicine and pediatrics specifically, although promising efforts by the American Academy of Pediatrics recently outline recommendations designed to better prepare pediatricians to take on a larger role in addressing mental health issues (Green et al., 2019). Second, although current psychological treatments within a medical context have demonstrated promising results, the reported treatment effects are generally small (Fisher et al., 2014). One reason for this could be the vast heterogeneity in symptom presentation within pediatric samples with comorbid medical conditions, where treatments to date have primarily focused on a select subset of physical and mental symptomatology. In addition to limiting the generalizability of treatment, this focus on treating either physical or psychological symptoms is likely insufficient given the frequency of co-occurring physical and mental health issues (Reigada et al., 2008). These limitations make transdiagnostic approaches like the UP-C/A particularly appealing within pediatric and integrated care settings.

Adaptation of the Unified Protocols to Pediatric Health

A biopsychosocial approach to chronic illness takes an interdisciplinary perspective, considering the complex interaction between biological, psychological, and socioenvironmental factors that contribute to the onset and maintenance of a disease (Gatchel et al., 2007). From this viewpoint, diseases traditionally considered primarily through a biological lens become multidimensional constructs where both somatic and affective facets are taken into consideration when formulating a treatment strategy. How someone experiences pain, for example, is strongly influenced by affective states (Vinall et al., 2016). Research investigating the biopsychosocial processes of chronic diseases has found evidence supporting several common psychological mechanisms, including neurobiological processes and emotion regulation that underlie both physical and emotional symptomatology (Koechlin et al, 2018; Vinall et al., 2016).

Indeed, several traditional psychological therapies have been adapted to assist in the treatment of specific medical illnesses such as asthma (Deshmukh et al., 2007) and diabetes (Li et al., 2017) and issues with chronic pain (Eccleston et al., 2014). More recently, however, several transdiagnostic approaches to treating comorbid somatic and psychiatric symptoms have been developed, with the most promising research surrounding the treatment of chronic pain (Reigada et al., 2008; Weersing et al., 2012). The UP-A has also been successfully adapted to address chronic pain issues (Allen et al., 2012). The Unified Protocol for the Treatment of Emotions in Youth with Pain (UP-YP) differs from other transdiagnostic approaches in several key areas. First, it differs from a theoretical perspective in that it moves beyond conventional cognitive-behavioral approaches and instead emphasizes the identification and modification of maladaptive emotion regulation patterns connected with the experience of pain. Here the primary aim is teaching more adaptive emotion regulation strategies that can be applied across a variety of situations and settings that may be applied to cope with pain, anger, anxiety, depression, or other emotions. Second, as with other UP approaches, managing emotional distress and teaching adaptive emotion regulation strategies remains a consistent target and can therefore be applied more flexibly across a variety of clinical presentations.

The UP-YP was designed as a modular intervention protocol, adapted from UP-A and UP-C interventions to address both pain and emotion dysregulation (Allen et al., 2012). Treatment consists of eight to 21 50-minute sessions across six months. The five primary modules within UP-YP consist of (1) psychoeducation about emotions and pain; (2) awareness of emotions and pain; (3) flexibility in thinking; (4) modifying emotion-driven behaviors through exposures; and (5) treatment review and relapse prevention. Additionally, there are several optional modules: (1) building and keeping motivation; (2) keeping safe (for adolescents displaying suicidal ideation); and (3) parenting emotional adolescents with pain.

Research and Intervention Recommendations

Empirical support for UP-YP has been limited to date, as this approach has yet to be tested in a randomized controlled trial. However, in a pilot study, Allen et al. (2010) found that adolescents with a chronic pain disorder and comorbid anxiety or depressive symptoms demonstrated improvements in symptoms of anxiety and depression as well as improvements in functional disability. These results provide initial support for the potential of a comprehensive transdiagnostic treatment protocol capable of addressing both physical discomfort and emotional distress. More importantly, initial data suggest the inclusion of emotion regulation skills in addition to cognitive-behavioral strategies may be valuable when providing treatment with both physical and emotional components. Future research should emphasize the continued evaluation of UP-YP across a variety of pain disorders and clinical presentations, as well as investigating its clinical utility in treating other chronic health conditions common in children.

Barriers

While approaching pediatric illness from a transdiagnostic perspective has demonstrated clinical utility in improving treatment outcomes, there are still a number of obstacles that need to be addressed. First, as was described earlier, behavioral health concerns are often not recognized by primary care providers (Barbui & Tansella, 2006), and parents are often hesitant to discuss any concerns about their child's mental health with their pediatrician (Briggs-Gowan et al., 2000). Second, discussing the possibility of psychological causes for pain or discomfort with clients is often unwelcome, as there is a greater stigma associated with psychological as opposed to physical health concerns (Wakefield et al., 2018). These two obstacles will continue to prove challenging until there is a better representation of mental health professionals within primary care settings. The recognition of the inextricable link between pediatric illnesses and settings also underlies the limited research on the use of transdiagnostic approaches across the variety of pediatric conditions. While somatic and chronic pain concerns are the most logical fits in many ways, further use of transdiagnostic approaches in pediatric settings may also spur further research with other chronic medical conditions.

Case Example

Mateo, a 14-year-old Hispanic male, was referred to us by his primary care physician due to concerns about ongoing unexplained gastrointestinal pain. Mateo reported that his stomach hurt nearly every day, and he would get sick to the point where he "couldn't think." He stated that the pain was "constant" but reported no vomiting, constipation, or diarrhea. In addition to his stomach pain, Mateo was already receiving treatment for fibromyalgia about one year prior to his referral. Mateo often reported widespread joint pain, though his joints were never red or swollen, along with chronic fatigue and difficulties sleeping. Mateo's symptoms had shown no improvement since he began taking tramadol following his diagnosis, and he had missed several days of school as a result of his significant pain symptoms.

Mateo also reported experiencing symptoms of depression and anxiety that began shortly after his initial pain symptoms. He described feeling depressed almost daily, lacking interest in most activities apart from playing video games after school, struggling to fall asleep, having difficulty concentrating, and feeling irritated by his family and friends. Although Mateo denied having active thoughts of self-harm or suicide, he mentioned feeling like a burden to his family and stated that their lives would "be easier without me."

INTEGRATIVE ASSESSMENT AND CASE CONCEPTUALIZATION

A pediatric psychologist reviewed Mateo's complete medical and psychological history. After a biopsychosocial assessment, it was concluded that while his fibromyalgia likely initiated his joint pain, fatigue, and sleep issues, his reports of stomach pain were not associated with his diagnosis and were likely psychological. Mateo was also presenting with symptoms of depression. However, since his fibromyalgia was likely the primary trigger of his depressive symptoms he was diagnosed with depressive disorder due to another medical condition (F06.31) with depressive features. As Mateo's symptoms were connected both behaviorally and emotionally, the UP-YP protocol was used to address his dysregulated emotional responses to pain by exploring the bidirectional relationship between his physical and emotional symptoms.

TREATMENT OVERVIEW

Module 1: Psychoeducation About Emotions and Pain. Mateo participated in a total of 18 50-minute sessions over a six-month period. The first 12 sessions were provided weekly, with the final six occurring biweekly as Mateo began to demonstrate proficiency in skills taught throughout therapy as well as a reduction in symptoms. Therapy began by providing Mateo with basic psychoeducation about the relationship between emotions and pain responses. During this module, Mateo was encouraged to consider situations where his emotional responses to pain had been functional as well as examples that had been dysfunctional. He was able to recognize how the anxiety he experienced after he sprained his ankle was functional in helping him avoid vigorous activity until his ankle had healed. Conversely, he was able to identify that whenever he experienced pain, he would feel down and angry and often isolated himself from his friends and family. In addition to identifying instances where his pain influenced his emotions, Mateo was also encouraged to monitor his mood for several weeks and noticed that his negative moods seemed to trigger his pain in some instances.

The additional optional module, "Parenting Emotional Adolescents with Pain," was also included in Mateo's treatment plan. Mateo's parents attended parallel sessions with Mateo to receive psychoeducation about pain, as well as to learn how to support Mateo in subsequent interventions. This also provided his parents the opportunity to receive support and encouragement in managing challenging situations with Mateo and helped to promote school attendance and setting consistent expectations for Mateo with his pain.

Module 2: Awareness of Emotions and Pain. In the second module, Mateo was taught skills to help him become more aware of his emotional responses to pain. In session, he was asked to notice both bodily sensations that triggered pain and his emotional responses to that pain. Mateo had difficulty with these exercises and would often stop as soon as he experienced discomfort and was also very hesitant to accept or express his emotions. Once this pattern of emotional avoidance was identified, Mateo was encouraged to identify examples of times he had attempted to control, avoid, or escape from his emotions and worked with his therapist to identify a pattern in his behavior.

Module 3: Flexibility in Thinking. Throughout the third module, Mateo worked to develop flexibility in thinking skills. As he worked to apply CLUES skills, he was able to look at his thoughts related to his fibromyalgia and associated chronic pain, such as "I'll never be allowed to leave my parents' house if I have chronic pain" and "I am a burden on my family." Using detective thinking, he was able to identify the thinking trap of "Jumping to Conclusions" for these scenarios. He was also able to identify situations where those thoughts were not accurate. For example, Mateo's parents were anxious about not being able to care for him when he left home; however, they frequently allowed him to attend after-school events alone and had already agreed to let him spend a long weekend at his friend's lake cabin out of town.

Module 4: Modifying Emotion-Driven Behaviors Through Exposure. Over the course of treatment, it became clear that Mateo's difficulty expressing his feelings, inability to tolerate frustration and anger, and feelings of sadness triggered by pain all contributed to a dysfunctional mood–pain relationship. These three issues were identified as primary targets for change because they directly resulted in avoidance of emotion and pain-related triggers, further exacerbating this dysfunctional mood–pain relationship. As a result, the focus of the fourth module was exposure and inhibitory learning regarding management of uncomfortable emotion states (such as those experienced when dealing with chronic pain). This effort included having Mateo identify uncomfortable emotion states when they occur and observe these emotions, at least briefly, before taking avoidant or maladaptive approach-oriented actions to reduce or eliminate discomfort. For example, Mateo would often leave school early if he experienced pain, or not go to school at all. To address this in Module 4, together with his parents, Mateo set goals related to increased attendance at school, even on days with mild pain, as a means of reducing avoidance of school due to fear of experiencing pain. This had several benefits, as it allowed Mateo to experience being able to engage in greater levels of activity, even if some pain was anticipated, while also minimizing the academic disruption that compounded his chronic pain, and promoting more time with friends. As a result, Mateo reported increases in positive behaviors with friends that both improved his mood and gave him additional examples for his detective thinking about being able to gain some level of independence from his family. During this module, Mateo also worked to identify other situations that he avoided due to pain. Mateo was able to return to some of the body scanning exercises from Module 2 and attempt them even while experiencing pain as a means of pausing in an exposure situation, noticing his bodily sensations, and continuing to engage in that situation, where possible. Over time, Mateo became more comfortable with both persisting in previously avoided activities despite some pain and increasingly noticed that the pain would typically subside over time. As his pain symptoms and level of engagement improved, his mood symptoms continued to improve as well.

Module 5: Treatment Review and Relapse Prevention. Over the course of treatment, Mateo demonstrated improvement in several areas of functioning. His self-reported symptoms of depression improved, while somatization decreased over the course of treatment. These changes were especially noteworthy given that Mateo's level of pain was highly variable throughout treatment due to the nature of his condition. The optional module of "Keeping Safe" (for adolescents displaying suicidal ideation) was included as a preventive measure in case his thoughts of burdensomeness developed into self-harm thoughts or behaviors. However, fortunately, his behavioral engagement helped support an improved mood and decreased feelings of burdensomeness. Mateo was able to verbalize this himself as he reflected on his course of treatment and was able to identify key behaviors to engage in (e.g., attending school despite pain) to reduce future relapse.

PEDIATRIC HEALTH SETTINGS

Pediatric settings can have a broad definition—from inpatient consultation and liaison services to outpatient ambulatory care. This chapter will focus primarily on the use of transdiagnostic protocols in integrated primary health care settings, as that is not only where the majority of behavioral health care occurs (even if not always discussed) but also a reliable location for preventive health engagement for children (Briggs et al., 2016). This is also consistent with existing research on the use of the UP-C/A in pediatric settings, as previous work has focused heavily on primary care (Weersing et al., 2017).

Applying transdiagnostic principles within primary care settings does not differ significantly from specialty care settings like those reviewed above—whether it is medical or psychological in nature. The biggest differences in primary care settings tend to be in terms of acuity (lower) and treatment intensity (brief, less intense, but more time sensitive). One of the most common models of integrated primary care speaks to the idea of high-volume services that are routine and accessible (Reiter et al., 2017). As such, the focus on lower treatment intensity in both frequency and duration, complemented by generally lower acuity, requires an adaptation of the UP-C/A that still recognizes the value inherent within more specialized care settings and modalities.

Adapting the UP-C/A to Pediatric Settings

Adaptations of the UP-C/A to pediatric settings are limited, but a similar transdiagnostic approach has been utilized by Weersing et al. (2017) in the form of Brief Behavioral Therapy (BBT). One key adaptation of BBT was a focus on simplicity—seeking to reduce barriers for training and fidelity in simplifying therapeutic objectives, as well as seeking to streamline interventions for a shorter-duration setting. This also lends itself to a modular design, whereby key themes of transdiagnostic treatments can be lifted out and placed independently in an intervention setting. This is also particularly attractive given the diversity of presenting concerns seen in a pediatric environment.

Weersing et al. (2017) found that their transdiagnostic adaptation yielded positive findings in symptom reduction and functioning across a sample of diverse youth using an eight- to 12-session adaptation delivered in primary care. This offers promise for future research, although it is still similar in length to the administration of UP-A seen in specialty care settings. The idea of being able to evaluate particular modules that could be given in various sequences is consistent with newer work in dissemination science (c.f. Collins, 2018) as well as even further reduction in complexity and brevity. It should be noted that many primary care behavioral health interventions are envisioned as "single shot" or very limited (e.g., less than four visits) protocols (c.f. the Multifaceted Diabetes and Depression Program [MDDP] and Prolonged Exposure for Primary Care [PE-PC]; Cigrang et al., 2015; Ell et al., 2010). While there has been some recognition that pediatric settings offer some unique challenges in integrated care with lack of established training programs (Landoll et al., 2019), there is still a gap in understanding how much intervention is too much or too little, so it is important to proceed with caution in oversimplifying transdiagnostic approaches.

Nevertheless, the focus on core dysfunctions and the adaptable structure of the UP-C (Ehrenreich-May et al., 2017) show promise for potential adaptations of briefer duration. For example, the CLUES paradigm in Emotion Detectives could be adapted for primary care in a standalone context. Although not empirically tested, this would involve emotional awareness (Consider How I Feel), cognitive appraisal and disputation (Look at My Thoughts and Use Detective Thinking), emotional exposure (Experience My Fears and Feelings), and relapse prevention (Stay Happy and Healthy). Clinicians interested in applying these transdiagnostic approaches from the UP-C/A in a pediatric setting might consider how they may be able to pull a single concept into a brief visit with a child in hopes of establishing more regular care. Alternatively, brief group treatments centered around a single element of the CLUES skills could decrease the total number of appointments by over 50% from the standard UP-A protocol. This may help to address a key barrier in this setting in that children are often seen in discrete episodes of care. A more discrete modular focus may be able to promote continuity.

Clinicians can also leverage other team members in this integrated care setting to reinforce the concepts and principles taught using a transdiagnostic approach. For example, this might mean teaching a pediatrician to inquire about a child's use of CLUES skills or collaborating on shared exposures (e.g., a child who has a fear of needle sticks and thus avoids blood sugar checks as part of their diabetes treatment regimen). This team-based approach to care can help reinforce the transdiagnostic nature of the UP-C/A, as the principles of emotional awareness, labeling, and experiential non-avoidance can be applied across different contexts and settings.

CONCLUSION

Pediatric health conditions and settings are excellent targets for use of transdiagnostic treatments, the UP-C/A in particular. Pediatric conditions tend to share a high degree of comorbidity with behavioral health disorders, and somatic symptoms in childhood are commonplace. Furthermore, the focus on underlying core processes in the UP-C/A can help with addressing a more comprehensive biopsychosocial view of a child's health. Nevertheless, existing research is limited primarily to chronic pain and would benefit from exploration of other chronic health concerns (e.g., diabetes).

In regard to pediatric settings, modular adaptations of the UP-C/A may be particularly helpful in these settings as it provides flexibility in implementation and targets a broader range of symptoms than other evidence-based treatments. Indeed, despite being a burgeoning area of study, there have already been promising results for transdiagnostic treatments within schools and primary care settings (García-Escalera et al., 2019; Weersing et al., 2017). While these initial findings are promising, several issues must be considered within these settings, including educating and involving stakeholders and reducing the burden of screening and referral for the multidisciplinary team members who may be unfamiliar with behavioral health concerns. Additionally, in primary care settings, it is important to recognize that there may be more variability in acuity and that parents may also be less likely to disclose behavioral health concerns. As such, continuing to implement adaptations in primary care that can help to normalize behavioral health is of critical importance.

Tip Sheet for Using UP-C and UP-A in Pediatric Illnesses and Settings

✓ **Why use UP-C and UP-A with pediatric health conditions?**
- UP-C and UP-A treatments are flexible across diagnoses and sensitive to subclinical symptoms.
- Stress is comorbid with sensitivity to pain and emotional regulation difficulties.
- Physical complaints with unknown origin are common in childhood.
- Research suggests behavioral health interventions improve physical health outcomes.
- Use of these treatments allows for a biopsychosocial approach to chronic illness using interdisciplinary perspectives.

✓ **How do I adapt UP-C and UP-A to chronic pediatric health conditions?**
- Use the UP-YP modules as an example (Allen et al., 2012) for dissemination:
  - Provide psychoeducation about emotions and physical symptoms
  - Identify function of physical symptoms
  - Teach flexibility in thinking skills
  - Use exposure to change emotion-driven behaviors
  - Review treatment progress
  - Prepare for relapse
  o As skills are developed, decrease session frequency.

✓ **Why use UP-C and UP-A in pediatric health settings?**
- Pediatric health settings offer access to care for youth who are unable to seek care in traditional behavioral health settings.
- UP-C/A allows for symptom heterogeneity.
- Primary care is a great setting for transdiagnostic treatments.
- Treatment fidelity is easier by reducing therapeutic objectives.

✓ **How do I use UP-C and UP-A in pediatric primary care?**
- Adapt the treatments to shorter frequency and duration and less acute symptoms.
- Leverage medical team members by providing education about treatment concepts.
- Use single components of UP-C and UP-A—for example, the Look at My Thoughts and Use Detective Thinking components of the Emotion Detectives treatment protocol (Ehrenreich-May et al., 2017).

✓ **What challenges might come up when using UP-C and UP-A with diverse settings and conditions?**
- Behavioral health concerns may not be recognized by medical professionals.
- Parents may not mention behavioral health symptoms to medical professionals.
- Youth may struggle to identify their psychological symptoms over medical symptoms.
- Pediatric health settings may provide less continuity in care.
- All members of the interdisciplinary team must be involved in treatment planning.

REFERENCES

Allen, K. B., Benningfield, M., & Blackford, J. U. (2020). Childhood anxiety: If we know so much, why are we doing so little? *JAMA Psychiatry, 77*(9), 887–888.

Allen, L. B., Tsao, J. C. I., Seidman, L. C., Ehrenreich-May, J., & Zeltzer, L. K. (2012). A unified, transdiagnostic treatment for adolescents with chronic pain and comorbid anxiety and depression. *Cognitive and Behavioral Practice, 19*(1), 56–67.

Allen, L. B., Tsao, J. C. I., Zeltzer, L. K., Ehrenreich-May, J. T., & Barlow, D. H. (2010). *Unified Protocol for Treatment of Emotions in Youth with Pain (UP-YP)*. Pediatric Pain Program, UCLA.

Barbui, C., & Tansella, M. (2006). Identification and management of depression in primary care settings: A meta-review of evidence. *Epidemiology and Psychiatric Sciences, 15*(4), 276–283.

Barlow, D. H., Farchione, T. J., Fairholme, C. P., Ellard, K. K., Boisseau, C. L., Allen, L. B., & Ehrenreich-May, J. (2011). *Unified protocol for transdiagnostic treatment of emotional disorders: Therapist guide*. Oxford University Press.

Boisseau, C. L., Farchione, T. J., Fairholme, C. P., Ellard, K. K., & Barlow, D. H. (2010). The development of the unified protocol for the transdiagnostic treatment of emotional disorders: A case study. *Cognitive and Behavioral Practice, 17*(1), 102–113.

Briggs, R. D., German, M., Schrag Hershberg, R., Cirilli, C., Crawford, D. E., & Racine, A. D. (2016). Integrated pediatric behavioral health: Implications for training and intervention models. *Professional Psychology: Research and Practice, 47*(4), 312–319.

Briggs-Gowan, M. J., Horowitz, S. M., Schwab-Stone, M. E., Leventhal, J. M., & Leaf, P. J. (2000). Mental health in pediatric settings: Distribution of disorders and factors related to service use. *Journal of the American Academy of Child & Adolescent Psychiatry, 39*, 841–849.

Butler, A., Lieshout, R. J. V., Lipman, E. L., MacMillan, H. L., Gonzalez, A., Gorter, J. W., Georgiades, K., Speechley, K. N., Boyle, M. H., & Ferro, M. A. (2018). Mental disorder in children with physical conditions: A pilot study. *BMJ Open, 8*, e019011.

Canning, E. H., Hanser, S. B., Shade, K. A., & Boyce, W. T. (1992). Mental disorders in chronically ill children: Parent–child discrepancy and physician identification. *Pediatrics, 90*(5), 692–696.

Cigrang, J. A., Rauch, S. A., Mintz, J., Brundige, A. R., Avila, L. L., Bryan, C. J., Goodie, J. L., & Peterson, A. L. (2015). Treatment of active duty military with PTSD in primary care: A follow-up report. *Journal of Anxiety Disorders, 36*, 110–114 .

Cleave, J. V., Gortmaker, S. L., & Perrin, J. M. (2010). Dynamics of obesity and chronic health conditions among children and youth. *Journal of the American Medical Association, 303*(7), 623–630.

Collins, L. M. (2018). *Optimization of behavioral, biobehavioral, and biomedical interventions: The Multiphase Optimization Strategy (MOST)*. Springer International Publishing.

Deshmukh, V. M., Toelle, B. G., Usherwood, T., O'Grady, B., & Jenkins, C. R. (2007). Anxiety, panic and adult asthma: A cognitive-behavioral perspective. *Respiratory Medicine, 101*(2), 194–202.

Eccleston, C., Palermo, T. M., Williams, A. C. de C., Holley, A. L., Morley, S., Fisher, E., & Law, E. (2014). Psychological therapies for the management of chronic and recurrent pain in children and adolescents. *Cochrane Database of Systematic Reviews, 5,* CD003968.

Ehrenreich-May, J., Kennedy, S. M., Sherman, J. A., Bilek, E. L., Buzzella, B. A., Bennett, S. M., & Barlow, D. H. (2017). *Unified protocols for transdiagnostic treatment of emotional disorders in children and adolescents: Therapist guide.* Oxford University Press.

Ell, K., Katon, W., Xie, B., Lee, P. J., Kapetanovic, S., Guterman, J., & Chou, C. P. (2010). Collaborative care management of major depression among low-income, predominantly Hispanic subjects with diabetes: A randomized controlled trial. *Diabetes Care, 33*(4), 706–713.

Fisher, E., Heathcote, L., Palermo, T. M., de C. Williams, A. C., Lau, J., & Eccleston, C. (2014). Systematic review and meta-analysis of psychological therapies for children with chronic pain. *Journal of Pediatric Psychology, 39*(8), 763–782.

García-Escalera, J. Chorot, P., Sandín, B., Ehrenreich-May, J., Prieto, A., & Valiente, R. M. (2019). An open trial applying the unified protocol for transdiagnostic treatment of emotional disorders in adolescents (UP-A) adapted as a school-based prevention program. *Child & Youth Care Forum, 48*(1), 29–53.

Gatchel, R. J., Peng, Y. B., Peters, M. L., Fuchs, P. N., & Turk, D. C. (2007). The biopsychosocial approach to chronic pain: Scientific advances and future directions. *Psychological Bulletin, 133*(4), 581–624.

Green, C. M., Foy, J. M., Earls, M. F., & Committee on Psychosocial Aspects of Child and Family Health. (2019). Achieving the pediatric mental health competencies. *Pediatrics, 144*(5), e20192758.

Gureje, O., Simon, G. E., & Von Korff, M. (2001). A cross-national study of the course of persistent pain in primary care. *Pain, 92*(1–2), 195–200.

Hughes, A. A., Lourea-Waddell, B., & Kendall, P. C. (2008). Somatic complaints in children with anxiety disorders and their unique prediction of poorer academic performance. *Child Psychiatry and Human Development, 39*(2), 211–220.

Koechlin, H., Coakley, R., Schechter, N., Werner, C., & Kossowsky, J. (2018). The role of emotion regulation in chronic pain: A systematic literature review. *Journal of Psychosomatic Research, 107,* 38–45.

Kroenke, K., & Swindle, R. (2000). Cognitive-behavioral therapy for somatization and symptom syndromes: A critical review of controlled clinical trials. *Psychotherapy and Psychosomatics, 69*(4), 205–215.

Landoll, R. R., Elmore, C. A., Weiss, A. F., & Garza, J. A. (2019). Training issues in pediatric psychology. In R. D. Friedberg & J. K. Paternostro (Eds.), *Handbook of cognitive behavioral therapy for pediatric medical conditions* (pp. 419–431). Springer.

Li, C., Xu, D., Hu, M., Tan, Y., Zhang, P., Li, G., & Chen, L. (2017). A systematic review and meta-analysis of randomized controlled trials of cognitive behavior therapy for patients with diabetes and depression. *Journal of Psychosomatic Research, 95,* 44–54.

Masia Warner, C., Reigada, L. C., Fisher, P. H., Saborsky, A. L., & Benkov, K. J. (2009). CBT for anxiety and associated somatic complaints in pediatric medical settings: An open pilot study. *Journal of Clinical Psychology in Medical Settings, 16*(2), 169–177.

Mojtabai, R., Olfson, M., & Han, B. (2016). National trends in the prevalence and treatment of depression in adolescents and young adults. *Pediatrics, 138*(6), e20161878.

Quach, J., & Barnett, T. (2015). Impact of chronic illness timing and persistence at school entry on child and parent outcomes: Australian longitudinal study. *Academic Pediatrics, 15*(1), 89–95.

Rapee, R. M., Schniering, C. A., & Hudson, J. L. (2009). Anxiety disorders during childhood and adolescence: Origins and treatment. *Annual Review of Clinical Psychology, 5*, 311–341.

Reigada, L. C., Fisher, P. H., Cutler, C., & Warner, C. M. (2008). An innovative treatment approach for children with anxiety disorders and medically unexplained somatic complaints. *Cognitive and Behavioral Practice, 15*(2), 140–147.

Reiter, J. T., Dobmeyer, A. C., & Hunter, C. L. (2017). The primary care behavioral health (PCBH) model: An overview and operational definition. *Journal of Clinical Psychology in Medical Settings, 25*, 109–126.

Vinall, J., Pavlova, M., Asmundson, G. J. G., Rasic, N., & Noel, M. (2016). Mental health comorbidities in pediatric chronic pain: A narrative review of epidemiology, models, neurobiological mechanisms and treatment. *Children, 3*(4), 40.

Vogel, M. E., Kanzler, K. E., Aikens, J. E., & Goodie, J. L. (2017). Integration of behavioral health and primary care: Current knowledge and future directions. *Journal of Behavioral Medicine, 40*(1), 69–84.

Wakefield, E. O., Zempsky, W. T., Puhl, R. M., & Litt, M. D. (2018). Conceptualizing pain-related stigma in adolescent chronic pain: A literature review and preliminary focus group findings. *Pain Reports, 3*(Suppl. 1), e679.

Weersing, V. R., Brent, D. A., Rozenman, M. S., Aracello Gonzalez, M. J., Dickerson, J. F., Lynch, F. L., Porta, G, & Iyengar, S. (2017). Brief behavioral therapy for pediatric anxiety and depression in primary care: A randomized clinical trial. *JAMA Psychiatry, 74*(6), 571–578.

Weersing, V. R., Rozenman, M. S., Maher-Bridge, M., & Campo, J. V. (2012). Anxiety, depression, and somatic distress: Developing a transdiagnostic internalizing toolbox for pediatric practice. *Cognitive and Behavioral Practice, 19*(1), 68–82.

Yorke, J., Fleming, S. L., & Shuldham, C. (2007). Psychological interventions for adults with asthma: A systematic review. *Respiratory Medicine, 101*(1), 1–14.

PART 3

Adapting the UP-C and UP-A to Different Treatment Settings

10

Stepped Care and Telehealth Delivery

JUDY H. HONG, ALISON SALLOUM, JAFAR BAKHSHAIE,
THANH T. TRUONG, JILL EHRENREICH-MAY,
AND ERIC A. STORCH ■

OVERVIEW OF STEPPED CARE AND TELEHEALTH DELIVERY

Service delivery models are needed to address barriers to youth receiving effective psychological treatment for depressive and anxiety disorders. Common barriers to treatment participation include cost, logistical issues (e.g., time, work demands, childcare, transportation), and stigma (Meredith et al., 2009; Salloum et al., 2016). Other barriers to accessing treatment are related to availability of trained clinicians (Bringewatt & Gershoff, 2010) and parent preferences to implement their own solutions to solve the child's problems (Thurston & Phares, 2008). A stepped care transdiagnostic treatment for children and adolescents with emotional problems, with an option for telehealth delivery, has the potential to address several of these treatment barriers. Stepped care models that require less clinician time, reduce provider costs, and allow more time for trained clinicians to provide care for clients requiring more intensive treatment. Stepped care models may also save time for clients, especially those who respond after the first step, thereby reducing treatment costs. Stigma of therapy may be decreased if stepped care models include steps that are not directed by the clinician, such as parent-led treatments, which may also help parents feel a sense of self-efficacy in helping their child. The purpose of this chapter is to illustrate how the Unified Protocols for Transdiagnostic Treatment of Emotional Disorders in Children and Adolescents (UP-C/A) has been adapted into a stepped care intervention (UP-C/A-SC) that may be delivered via telehealth.

STEPPED CARE INTERVENTIONS

Stepped care models are designed to be efficient, effective, accessible, and cost-effective personalized service delivery models that match the most appropriate dosage or the best type of treatment to the client's needs. Principles of stepped care models include the following:

1. The first step (intervention) should be the "least restrictive," usually meaning it requires less clinician time, is lower in cost, is less time-intensive, or is more convenient for the client.
2. The first step should be effective for a substantial number of clients.
3. Processes should be in place to monitor treatment progress and to support clear decision-making about when to "step up" to the next, more intensive treatment or "step down" to a less intensive treatment level or treatment termination (Bower & Gilbody, 2005).

Less time in the first step can be achieved in many ways, such as by having parents lead some of the sessions or having fewer sessions; however, first steps need to include active mechanisms of change so that a substantial number of clients respond to Step 1 and can end or lessen their involvement in treatment. There also should be clear decisional rules about when a client needs to step up or down based on degree of response. Clients who do not respond after the first step will step up to more intensive care, usually involving more clinician and client time. Stepped care models vary in terms of the number of steps (i.e., number of different types of treatment and/or dosages provided), types of treatment provided, ways to monitor treatment progress, and how the decision is made about when, or if, to step up to the next type of treatment.

While more research is needed on potential advantages and disadvantages of stepped care interventions, they are designed to lower costs and provide a first-line, least-restrictive treatment so that resources, such as trained clinician time and costs of treatment, are shifted to those needing more intensive care. In community mental health centers where there may be a waitlist for youth with emotional disorders to receive specialized treatment, a stepped care, transdiagnostic intervention may minimize wait times as clients can begin with the first-line treatment. As research on stepped care interventions with children and adolescents advances, more adaptive treatments can be provided to identify parent and child characteristics, prior to beginning treatment, in order to match children to the best level of care (e.g., step): Some children will be matched to start with Step 1, while others will go directly to more intensive steps based on need and clinical appropriateness. This type of method that matches care to intensity minimizes the number of children who are non-responders to Step 1.

TELEHEALTH DELIVERY

Telehealth utilizes technology to provide and improve clinical support to clients and to overcome geographical barriers to clients connecting to services (World Health Organization, 2010). Telehealth psychotherapy may be used to provide the first step of a stepped care intervention or, if clients find telehealth more accessible and convenient, all steps within a stepped care model. Stepped care models that include steps with limited clinician-directed therapy may be well suited for telehealth. Telehealth delivery can provide a convenient and accessible platform for children and their parents to receive treatment. For families with logistical barriers to attending in-office sessions or who live in rural areas or areas that do not have accessible, trained clinicians, telehealth can increase access to treatment. For parents struggling with financial costs of attending in-office sessions, telehealth can address barriers such as transportation or childcare costs for treatment attendance. Stigma may also be reduced via the use of telehealth delivery since clients do not need to go to a mental health professional's or a doctor's office but can receive care from their home.

Despite these advantages, there may be some reluctance for clinicians to provide treatment via telehealth, as well as some aspects that negatively impact care. For example, some clients do not like using a telehealth platform for therapy. Clinical assessment may be challenging for some clients, and connectivity issues can disrupt treatment provision. Clinicians who are concerned about the use of this platform for mental health services may benefit from observing telehealth sessions prior to implementation and/or receiving mentoring with a more senior telehealth clinician in order to address potential concerns related to building therapeutic alliance, comfort with technology, cost and confidentiality issues, and concerns related to effectiveness (McClellan et al., 2020).

Generally, studies using telehealth interventions to provide psychotherapy suggest that treatment outcomes and client satisfaction are comparable to traditional in-person psychotherapy (Backhaus et al., 2012), including for treatments that target depression (Berryhill et al., 2019a) and anxiety (Berryhill et al., 2019b), although studies with youth are still limited. Pilot and case studies delivering evidence-based interventions via telehealth to children with emotional disorders, including posttraumatic stress disorder (Stewart et al., 2017) and anxiety (Cooper-Vince et al., 2016; Storch et al., 2011), are promising. In summary, these findings support adaptation of UP-C/A to be delivered within a stepped care model using telehealth as a first step.

EFFICACY OF STEPPED CARE AND TELEHEALTH DELIVERY FOR CHILDHOOD EMOTIONAL DISORDERS

Research studies on stepped care interventions for children and adolescents have demonstrated efficacy and feasibility (Pettit et al., 2017; Rapee et al., 2017; Salloum et al., 2016b; van der Leeden et al., 2011), although these treatments target specific diagnoses. For example, in a study with 281 children (6 to 17 years old) comparing stepped care versus a standard in-office cognitive-behavioral therapy for pediatric anxiety, there was no difference in treatment outcomes, but clinician time was significantly less providing stepped care versus standard care. The first step consisted of brief phone support (four 30- to 40-minute phone sessions) to assist the parent and youth as they worked with empirically supported materials to decrease anxiety; 41% completed Step 1 and stepped down, and 59% stepped up to receive clinician-directed treatment (Rapee et al., 2017). Pilot studies in children (3 to 12 years old) with traumatic stress disorders testing parent-led, clinician-assisted treatment as a first step and standard, clinician-directed weekly trauma-focused treatment with children as the second step have demonstrated that approximately 75% of children responded to Step 1 (63% for the intent-to-treat group). Improvements in posttraumatic stress symptoms at post-assessment were comparable to those for standard weekly trauma-focused treatment, and both treatment time for clinician and parents and costs were lower with a stepped care intervention (Salloum et al., 2015, 2016b). While initial research on stepped care interventions for specific diagnostic categories in youth is promising, transdiagnostic stepped care models that address comorbidity, which is common in community samples, are needed. Accordingly, we adapted the UP-C/A to be delivered within a stepped care model using telehealth to address this need.

ADAPTATIONS TO UP-C AND UP-A FOR STEPPED CARE AND TELEHEALTH DELIVERY: UP-C/A-SC

Adaptations to the UP-C/A related to stepped care and telehealth model of delivery are discussed across five main categories: changes to the format, changes to delivery, changes to content, changes to materials (e.g., assessment methods), and changes related to the optional use of telehealth delivery.

Changes to the Format

In terms of format, the most important adaptation includes the use of a stepped approach to treatment (as discussed in the preceding section). Given that Rapee et al. (2017) found that the first two steps of psychotherapy provided the most improvement, while the third step of more psychotherapy did not demonstrate strong improvements, UP-C/A-SC was developed into a two-step model.

Other changes in format include changes in length. Compared to the UP-C with 15 sessions and the UP-A with a variable length of 12 to 21 sessions, UP-C/A-SC includes fewer therapy sessions (Kennedy et al., in press; Tonarely et al., in press). Specifically, for UP-C-SC, Step 1 (six or seven sessions) typically includes four joint parent–child telehealth sessions (Sessions 1, 2, 3, and 5 focus on psychoeducation, exposure, and acting opposite) as well as an optional, personalized intervention session (Session 7) for clients stepping down following Step 1. Two parent-directed telehealth support sessions (Sessions 4 and 6) are also conducted in this step to support home-based (parent and child only) sessions. Similar to Step 1, Step 2 of UP-C-SC (six sessions) also includes four joint parent–child sessions (Step 2 Sessions 1, 2, 3, and 5) and two parent-directed telehealth support (Step 2 Sessions 4 and 6) visits. During this step, however, the clinician is allowed to choose from the various UP-C-SC modalities to tailor the intervention to address the particular needs of the client (i.e., personalized targeting).

Unlike UP-C-SC, Step 1 of UP-A-SC typically includes up to six sessions with adolescents with no significant parent coaching or parent-led sessions (Tonarely et al., in press). On the other hand, similar to UP-C-SC, Step 1 of UP-A-SC comprises a standardized sequence of intervention components (Sessions 1 to 5 focused on psychoeducation, exposure, awareness, and acting opposite, and a sixth flex session). Further, during Step 2 of UP-A-SC (six sessions), clinicians are also free to select from a menu of the clinically appropriate, adolescent-focused interventions and to personalize treatment to address UP content most relevant to the adolescent's presenting problems. It is worth noting that as a consequence of the shorter duration of the therapy, UP-C/A-SC incorporates fewer UP-C/A components. Close to the end of Step 1 of UP-C/A-SC, the decision regarding stepping up or down the treatment is made (see the following for details).

Changes to Delivery

For UP-C-SC, the emphasis on a parent-led, clinician-assisted mode of therapy (particularly in Step 1) is one important delivery adaptation (Kennedy et al., in press). Parents are highly involved in assisting with exposure (e.g., Salloum et al., 2016b) and opposite action (Kennedy et al., in press) interventions both within and outside of the sessions. Parents are also expected to create a private and appropriate therapy environment and engage in troubleshooting in the case of technical difficulties in the context of an optional telehealth delivery method (see the following for details). This approach is particularly important during Step 1, in line with the general notion of cost-effective use as one of the goals of the stepped care method and to efficiently apportion clinician resources, allowing for more intensive treatment of high-complexity cases (Salloum et al., 2016b). It should also be mentioned that UP-A-SC does not include a parent-led delivery approach, as children may be more open to the parent-led treatment than adolescents.

Changes to Content

UP-C/A-SC is highly focused on specific content aspects of UP-C/A, including emotional and sensational awareness, exposure techniques, and opposite action strategies. Both UP-C-SC and UP-A-SC incorporate these components into Step 1. On the other hand, some components of UP-C/A are considered more elective in the stepped care context. For example, cognitive flexibility and detective thinking in UP-C-SC and cognitive reappraisal and problem solving in UP-A-SC are applied per the clinician's judgment, either in the context of a final (flex) session of Step 1 or as a part of Step 2 and in the service of a personalized therapy approach.

For UP-C-SC, in addition to some core UP-C/A components (e.g., emotional/sensational awareness, exposure exercises, and opposite action strategies), there is a strong focus on parent psychoeducation and pragmatic handling of parent-led, home-based interventions (Kennedy et al., in press). Even in Step 2, where there is a stronger emphasis on child-directed UP-C/A strategies, the clinician engages in substantial coaching, modeling, and supporting the parent for child-directed treatment delivery. Notably, during the UP-C-SC parent-only sessions, parents are instructed in the need for their active involvement in treatment and learn about skills needed to incorporate parent-led interventions (e.g., planning and supporting exposure) as well as addressing problematic emotional parenting behaviors that impede therapy progress (Ehrenreich-May et al., 2017).

The step-up or step-down process is another distinctive content adaptation made in UP-C/A-SC. This may be a collaborative decision-making process where the clinician helps the parent to reach a conclusion regarding stepping up or discontinuing treatment (Friedberg, 2017), although more directive and expert-based prescriptive approaches could also be used based on clinical necessity. When using collaborative decision-making, the clinician may choose to use a combination of pragmatic measures typically used for UP-C/A (e.g., Youth Top Problem Scale; Weisz et al., 2011), rating scales, and/or stakeholder preferences to engage the client and parent in a discussion about either stepping up or down at the end of Step 1. To assist with this collaborative decision-making process, we developed a Step Up/Step Down Questionnaire (Kennedy et al., in press) for use in UP-C-SC and UP-A-SC studies to assess clinician, parent, and child perception of improvement, satisfaction, and readiness to terminate treatment. Specifically, respondents are asked after Session 6 to answer questions concerning different indices of the client's progress by the end of Step 1, which are rated on a 5-point Likert scale (from 0 = *does not apply* to 4 = *true to a great extent*). The clinician version of the measure can also be used to assess the same constructs. The questionnaire was developed to be a brief, practical tool to easily use in the clinical setting with parents, children, and clinicians.

Changes to the Materials

In both UP-C-SC and UP-A-SC, relevant worksheets, forms, and figures from the full protocols are used in sessions for the purpose of illustrating concepts, engaging children in practice, and assigning homework. In the context of telehealth delivery, the workbook materials are available electronically (in addition to paper format) to clients and families. Clinicians may choose to screenshare worksheets, forms, and figures and ask children to complete them on the screen, and it is often helpful to illustrate UP concepts using multimedia and experiential exercises. Because of the individualized nature of the sessions, some material used in the UP-C group sessions (e.g., puzzle pieces to reinforce homework completion) are not utilized in UP-C-SC; instead, new activities to illustrate intervention components to parents and children are incorporated.

Changes Related to the Optional Use of Telehealth Delivery

The use of a videoconferencing platform is an optional but recommended delivery adaptation in UP-C/A-SC. The parent-only visits could be conducted by phone, if preferred or needed given poor connectivity. In a UP-C-SC pilot study, a secure telehealth platform (e.g., Vidyo) was used to provide four Step 1 sessions (50 minutes), which consisted of standardized sequenced UP-C/A components with the youth. When the two parent-only sessions occurred (30 to 40 minutes), parents were given the option of using video telesupport or phone-only. Given that there were geographical barriers, Step 2 (e.g., the same number of sessions but with a flexible, tailored clinical approach to address transdiagnostic problems) was also provided via Vidyo. The telehealth delivery approach has also been successfully used for UP-A-SC (Tonarely et al., 2020).

STEPPED CARE AND TELEHEALTH DELIVERY UP-C/ UP-A AS FIRST-LINE INTERVENTIONS, ADJUNCTIVE INTERVENTIONS, OR ALTERNATIVE INTERVENTIONS

The combination of UP-C/A in a stepped care format delivered through telehealth provides flexibility in application as a first-line intervention, an adjunct to traditional intervention, or an alternative intervention for children and adolescents with emotional disorders. This transdiagnostic protocol can target a wide range of emotional problems, including anxiety, depression, worry/rumination, adjustment, obsessive-compulsive symptoms, poor frustration tolerance, and disruptive behavior. Many children with emotional disorders may struggle to learn new behaviors in an unfamiliar environment, particularly when traveling to a clinic setting is difficult or physically and emotionally taxing. Using UP-C/A-SC to provide treatment in the home environment may result in improved learning and retention. Other clients who may benefit from this application as a first-line intervention include those who can only commit to a brief course of treatment and those with mild symptoms where brief treatment is sufficient. Other children who may only need brief treatment are those who successfully completed prior treatment and have a strong foundation of skills but experience a relapse in symptoms with life changes (e.g., going to school). There are other clients for whom traditional clinic treatment is preferred but is not an option due to cost or transportation barriers. An example would be a child with severe social anxiety, for whom the process of traveling to the clinic and interacting with others in person would

itself be part of the therapeutic intervention. While such a child would ideally receive clinic treatment as a first-line intervention, stepped care through telehealth
would be an appropriate alternative intervention to consider.

RELEVANT RESEARCH DATA PROVIDING EMPIRICAL SUPPORT FOR THE USE OF STEPPED CARE AND TELEHEALTH DELIVERY FOR UP-C OR UP-A

Empirical evidence regarding the delivery of UP-C/A using a stepped care and
telehealth delivery format is limited to date. However, existing research supports
the utility of this approach among children and adolescents with emotional
disorders. In a study focused on the development and implementation of UP-
C-SC delivered via telehealth, Kennedy et al. (in press) piloted a two-step UP-
C-SC treatment among three children with a wide range of emotional problems
(generalized anxiety, obsessive-compulsive, and adjustment symptoms).
Specifically, a stepped care adaptation of the UP-C-SC delivered via telehealth
consisting of the modifications described in this chapter was employed. Findings
provided preliminary support for the feasibility and acceptability of UP-C-SC for
a wide range of emotional disorders. Parents and children both reported being
satisfied with treatment, and participants generally showed a reduction in their
Top Problem ratings. Furthermore, in the context of the telehealth delivery, attendance and compliance were high across all participants.

Another study piloted UP-A-SC treatment among three adolescents with emotional problems using the UP-A-SC components described in this chapter. Results
demonstrated the feasibility and acceptability of this method, with significant improvement in anxiety, depression, and quality of life of the clients (Tonarely et al.,
in press). All sessions were successfully provided via telehealth delivery.

Collectively, these findings preliminarily suggest that UP-C/A-SC may be a
cost-effective transdiagnostic treatment for emotional disorders in children and
adolescents.

CASE EXAMPLE: STEP DOWN AFTER STEP 1 FOR UP-C-SC

Overview

The following case summary[1] illustrates the application of UP-C-SC in a client who
stepped down and ended treatment after the initial six sessions. Step 1 comprised
four, 50-minute joint child–parent sessions conducted using the Vidyo telehealth
platform. One session involved reviewing transdiagnostic, emotion-focused
psychoeducation, and three sessions focused on exposures to anger-provoking
situations and behavioral interventions. Additionally, two 30- to 40-minute
parent-only telehealth sessions were conducted to evaluate progress and determine next steps. Measures used were the Step Up/Step Down Questionnaire and

Top Problem ratings at baseline and treatment. Telehealth was chosen for this case due to convenience, as the family lived in a rural region of Texas that was nearly two hours from the authors' institution. The parent had several barriers to attending in-office treatment, including the burden of long travel time to the clinic (50 minutes each way), lack of childcare for siblings, and limited ability to take time off work to attend sessions.

Case Presentation

"Martha" was an eight-year-old Caucasian female who presented with her mother for treatment of disruptive mood dysregulation disorder. She displayed significant and impairing meltdowns, including anger/frustration and oppositionality, in home and in school. The meltdowns were exacerbated after Martha experienced bullying at school and when her four-year-old sister started to want to spend more time and play with her rather than stay by their mother's side as she did when she was younger. Martha would yell and refuse directives, causing class disruptions and changes in the family routine at home. At the time of evaluation, Martha would have meltdowns and, when corrected, expressed frustration and talked negatively about herself when she did not behave well. Top Problems were ranked from 0 to 8 (0 = *not at all a problem* and 8 = *very, very much a problem*). Top Problems identified by Martha and her mother included controlling frustration in school/home (Martha and mother ratings = 6/4), controlling meltdowns when corrected (5/4), and decreasing negative self-talk (6/4). Martha's ratings may have been higher than her mother's since Martha was very critical of herself and expressed remorse after she had meltdowns and, as she said, "acted bad." The mother sought treatment for her child because she felt she could not help her enough and also thought her behaviors seemed more extreme than what was typical for other children her age. However, the mother's ratings may have been in the middle (all 4s) since she had been helping her child with her meltdowns and moods and did not really see the problem as a "disorder"; rather, she thought her child just seemed to be "going through a bad phase."

Treatment

Step 1 comprised six sessions involving exposures centered on decreasing anger/frustration. In gradual succession, Martha was able to identify body clues, learned to tolerate strong physical sensations and refrained from behaviors to get rid of the sensations, and learned to respond to anger-provoking stimuli in more adaptive ways. The clinician took advantage of telehealth delivery to incorporate Martha's sibling into exposures. For example, Martha and her sibling were asked to engage in an activity that frequently led to disagreements and subsequent anger outbursts, and Martha was prompted to engage in opposite actions that she and the clinician had identified ahead of time. By the end of Step 1, reductions were noted in the frequency of write-ups in school, Martha's anger outbursts had decreased, and Martha had more days of earning privileges both at home and in school. In the fourth session, the clinician and Martha's mother discussed progress, problem-solving concerns, and ways in which Martha's mother could support her with new exposures for the following week. In Session 5, Martha was trained in body scanning to increase body and present-moment awareness. The clinician assisted Martha in updating her "My Emotion Ladder" worksheet and planned additional exposures. The sixth and final session of Step 1 involved evaluation of progress and discussion of whether Martha would step up or down in treatment. Martha's mother reported that Martha continued to struggle with meltdowns, but they were less intense. Psychoeducation was provided about meltdowns, how to reduce these behaviors, and how meltdowns would continue to lessen with consistent skills implementation. The clinician also collaborated with Martha's mother in deciding to step up or step down. The severity of Martha's Top Problems had decreased from her initial presentation as indicated by the following measures: controlling frustration in school/home (Martha's rating = 1/8; mother's rating = 1/8), controlling meltdowns when corrected (Martha's rating = 1/8; mother's rating = 2/8), and decreasing negative self-talk (Martha's rating 0/8; mother's rating = 0/8). All items from the Step Up/Step Down Questionnaire assessing clinician perception of client improvement were rated as being "True to a great extent" or "Mostly true" ("True to a great extent" indicates the highest degree of agreement with the statement). The Step Up/Step Down form indicated that all items rated by the parent were also "True to a great extent" or "Mostly true" as well, indicating high perceptions of improvement and satisfaction.

Martha decreased her anger outbursts, which resulted in an improved home environment and compliance with parental instruction. Martha also improved her overall school performance as she felt more comfortable expressing her feelings and understanding body clues. Based on ratings, examination of Step Up/Step Down forms, and qualitative feedback provided by the family, the recommendation to step down was made and accepted by the family. The clinician and family conducted a final seventh "flex session" to address the client's cognitive rigidity and frequent meltdowns, as well as an acknowledgment of progress and relapse prevention.

Should responses have indicated additional domains to target, Martha and her mother would have been stepped up for additional sessions personalized for her specific clinical needs, such as targeting emotion regulation and further exposure therapy.

POSSIBLE BARRIERS AND TROUBLESHOOTING IN USE OF STEPPED CARE

Since UP-C/A-SC is somewhat nontraditional in its implementation, a certain level of problem solving may be necessary, particularly at the beginning of treatment. A few common areas where troubleshooting may be helpful are rate of skills acquisition, treatment fidelity, challenges in deciding whether to step up or down, and logistical concerns.

In the beginning of treatment, specifically in the first six, brief sessions of Step 1, several concepts and skills are introduced. Depending on various factors (e.g., client and/or parent reading level, language barriers, parental level of psychopathology in the case of UP-C-SC), this rather rapid rate of skills introduction can be challenging for some families. It is the clinician's responsibility to make certain that these initial concepts are learned and the client and/or parent feels confident in these competencies. Extra time and material may be necessary to achieve this, but if skills acquisition continues to be a challenge, then additional sessions may be added in Step 1 to boost understanding. In addition, referring parents for their own treatment may be indicated, or the child may need to be stepped up immediately for a full course of UP-C/A should variables indicate attenuated likelihood of Step 1 response.

Treatment fidelity is a relevant concern with stepped care due to decreased amount of session time with clinicians. To manage this potential challenge, treatment agendas with detailed, written instructions are utilized, and clinicians should ensure consistent communication with the client and/or parent from week to week. For UP-C-SC, one of the biggest worries most parents have is their ability to effectively deliver learned skills outside of the session. The first six sessions are collaborative with the child, parent, and clinician together, but parent–clinician session are also scheduled regularly to keep progress on track and discuss any concerns the parent may have with delivering treatment material. It may also be helpful to remind the parent that as part of the step up/down process, if parents are having treatment delivery difficulties, the option to step up with an increase in clinician involvement and more instruction for parents is presented in the sixth or seventh session. It is also important for the therapist to normalize these concerns and be warm and supportive. Treatment fidelity should be monitored closely to ensure progress.

Another possible barrier involves the logistics of conducting the collaborative decision-making process after the sixth or seventh session of whether to step up or down. Various factors may be considered as part of this decision, including changes in symptom measures, client preference, family preference, clinician recommendation, and logistical barriers to stepping up or down. There is a risk that clients may receive more treatment and utilize more time and resources than necessary if they unnecessarily step up. On the other hand, clients may not receive adequate treatment if they inappropriately step down. This is a collective decision, and the clinician would typically present a recommendation based on the sources of information discussed earlier, but certainly more weight is placed on the client's and family's needs.

For telehealth treatment, common logistical concerns include finding appropriate therapy space in the home, technical difficulties, and insurance coverage. Establishing an appropriate space in the home for therapy is important for both the client and the parent. A suitable space is one that is private and free of distractions (e.g., electronic devices, toys, noise) and chaos, where the client can feel safe and is able to concentrate. This may be inside or outside of the home (e.g., empty room in a public library). Having a consistent, predetermined space for treatment may aid the client in establishing a routine. In addition to consistent space, holding sessions on the same day of the week and at the same time can aid the client in becoming accustomed to therapy and bolster compliance. Other challenges of the telehealth format include technical issues and difficulties exchanging documents (e.g., homework assignments, instructions). It may be helpful for clinicians to provide detailed, step-by-step instructions for connecting to sessions or even make an instructional video. If internet service is not reliable, a new therapy space may be necessary. Many of these issues are resolved quickly in the beginning of treatment with clinician help and once families become familiar with procedures.

Tip Sheet for Using UP-C/A-SC in Youth

✓ **Why use UP-C/A-SC?**
- It overcomes several common barriers to treatment, such as cost, time, geographical distance, waiting time for treatment, logistical issues, and stigma.
- Data support the feasibility of these protocols across emotional disorders, and they may be a good alternative to traditional, in-person, clinician-led treatment.

✓ **How does UP-C/A-SC differ from UP-C/A?**
- Changes to the format: fewer in-person sessions and shorter duration of treatment in general
- Changes to delivery: emphasis on parent-led sessions for UP-C-SC
- Changes to content: personalized, elective sessions; collaborative, client-tailored step up/step down process using the Step Up/Step Down Questionnaire
- Changes to materials: for UP-C-SC, strong focus on parent psychoeducation and pragmatic handling of parent-led, home-based interventions
- Optional use of telehealth delivery

✓ **Is UP-C/A-SC supported by research?**
- Although empirical support for stepped care UP-C/A is limited, existing studies support the model's feasibility and acceptability. A high degree of satisfaction has been reported from both parents and clients, with attendance and treatment compliance being high.

✓ **What are some troubleshooting tips for use of UP-C/A-SC?**
- Give parents a clear outline of the course of treatment and provide written materials ahead of time.
- Remind the parent that logistical concerns are common in the first few sessions and are to be expected.
- Use of a collaborative decision-making process to inform step up/down decisions can help to increase child and parent engagement in treatment and validate child and parent perceptions of progress.
- Regular and consistent monitoring of progress through assessments is essential for treatment fidelity and to ensure efficacy.

✓ **When is UP-C/A-SC not appropriate for a client?**
- If a child presents for treatment with more severe and/or impairing symptoms, it may be more effective to follow the full UP-A or UP-C treatment protocol.
- For some parents, their own distress or symptoms may interfere with their ability to effectively facilitate exposures with clinician coaching. In these cases, it may be best to conduct clinician-led exposures, including some sessions in the clinic.

NOTE

1. This case example is a clinical composite case comprising information from multiple child clients to illustrate the treatment course of UP-C-SC.

REFERENCES

Backhaus, A., Agha, Z., Maglione, M. L., Repp, A., Ross, B., Zuest, D., Rice-Thorp, N. M., Lohr, J., & Thorp, S. R. (2012). Videoconferencing psychotherapy: A systematic review. *Psychological Services, 9*(2), 111–131. doi:10.1037/a0027924

Berryhill, M. B., Culmer, N., Williams, N., Halli-Tierney, A., Betancourt, A., Roberts, H., & King, M. (2019a). Videoconferencing psychotherapy and depression: A systematic review. *Telemedicine Journal & E-Health, 25*(6), 435–446. doi:10.1089/tmj.2018.0058

Berryhill, M. B., Halli-Tierney, A., Culmer, N., Williams, N., Betancourt, A., King, M., & Ruggles, H. (2019b). Videoconferencing psychological therapy and anxiety: A systematic review. *Family Practice, 36*(1), 53–63. doi:10.1093/fampra/cmy072

Bower, P., & Gilbody, S. (2005). Stepped care in psychological therapies: Access, effectiveness and efficiency. Narrative literature review. *British Journal of Psychiatry, 186*, 11–17. doi:10.1192/bjp.186.1.11

Bringewatt, E. H., & Gershoff, E. T. (2010). Falling through the cracks: Gaps and barriers in the mental health system for America's disadvantaged children. *Children and Youth Services Review, 32*(10), 1291–1299. doi:10.1016/j.childyouth.2010.04.021

Cooper-Vince, C. E., Chou, T., Furr, J. M., Puliafico, A. C., & Comer, J. S. (2016). Videoteleconferencing early child anxiety treatment: A case study of the internet-delivered PCIT CALM (I-CALM) program. *Evidence-Based Practice in Child and Adolescent Mental Health, 1*(1), 24–39. doi:10.1080/23794925.2016.1191976

Ehrenreich-May, J., Kennedy, S. M., Sherman, J. A., Bilek, E. L., Buzzella, B. A., Bennett, S. M., & Barlow, D. H. (2017). *Unified protocols for transdiagnostic treatment of emotional disorders in children and adolescents: clinician guide.* Oxford University Press.

Friedberg, R. D. (2017). Care for a change? Tiered CBT for youth. *Journal of Rational-Emotive Cognitive-Behavior Therapy, 35*(3), 296–313.

Kennedy, S. M., Lanier, H., Salloum, A., Ehrenreich-May, J., & Storch, E. A. (in press). Development and implementation of a transdiagnostic, stepped-care approach to treating emotional disorders in children via telehealth. *Cognitive and Behavioral Practice.*

McClellan, M. J., Florell, D., Palmer, J., & Kidder, C. (2020). Clinician telehealth attitudes in a rural community mental health center setting. *Journal of Rural Mental Health, 44*(1), 62–73. doi:10.1037/rmh0000127

Meredith, L. S., Stein, B. D., Paddock, S. M., Jaycox, L. H., Quinn, V. P., Chandra, A., & Burnam, A. (2009). Perceived barriers to treatment for adolescent depression. *Medical Care, 47*(6), 677–685. doi:10.1097/MLR.0b013e318190d46b

Pettit, J. W., Rey, Y., Bechor, M., Melendez, R., Vaclavik, D., Buitron, V., Bar-Haim, Y., Pine, D. S., & Silverman, W. K. (2017). Can less be more? Open trial of a stepped care approach for child and adolescent anxiety disorders. *Journal of Anxiety Disorders, 51*, 7–13. doi:10.1016/j.janxdis.2017.08.004

Rapee, R. M., Lyneham, H. J., Wuthrich, V., Chatterton, M. L., Hudson, J. L., Kangas, M., & Mihalopoulos, C. (2017). Comparison of stepped care delivery against a single, empirically validated cognitive-behavioral therapy program for youth with anxiety: A randomized clinical trial. *Journal of the American Academy of Child & Adolescent Psychiatry, 56*(10), 841–848. doi:10.1016/j.jaac.2017.08.001

Salloum, A., Johnco, C., Lewin, A. B., McBride, N. M., & Storch, E. A. (2016a). Barriers to access and participation in community mental health treatment for anxious children. *Journal of Affective Disorders, 196*, 54–61. doi:10.1016/j.jad.2016.02.026

Salloum, A., Small, B. J., Robst, J., Scheeringa, M. S., Cohen, J. A., & Storch, E. A. (2015). Stepped and standard care for childhood trauma: A pilot randomized clinical trial. *Research on Social Work Practice, 27*(6), 653–663. doi:10.1177/1049731515601898

Salloum, A., Wang, W., Robst, J., Murphy, T. K., Scheeringa, M. S., Cohen, J. A., & Storch, E. A. (2016b). Stepped care versus standard trauma-focused cognitive behavioral therapy for young children. *Journal of Child Psychology and Psychiatry, 57*(5), 614–622. doi:10.1111/jcpp.12471

Stewart, R. W., Orengo-Aguayo, R. E., Cohen, J. A., Mannarino, A. P., & de Arellano, M. A. (2017). A pilot study of trauma-focused cognitive-behavioral therapy delivered via telehealth technology. *Child Maltreatment, 22*(4), 324–333. doi:10.1177/1077559517725403

Storch, E. A., Caporino, N. E., Morgan, J. R., Lewin, A. B., Rojas, A., Brauer, L., Larson, M. J., & Murphy, T. K. (2011). Preliminary investigation of web-camera delivered cognitive-behavioral therapy for youth with obsessive-compulsive disorder. *Psychiatry Research, 189*(3), 407–412. doi:10.1016/j.psychres.2011.05.047

Thurston, I. B., & Phares, V. (2008). Mental health service utilization among African American and Caucasian mothers and fathers. *Journal of Consulting and Clinical Psychology, 76*(6), 1058–1067. doi:10.1037/a0014007

Tonarely, N. A., Lanier, H., Salloum, A., Ehrenreich-May, J., & Storch, E. A. (In press). Tailoring the unified protocol for adolescents for a stepped-care approach: Case exemplars. *Journal of Cognitive Psychotherapy.*

van der Leeden, A. J., van Widenfelt, B. M., van der Leeden, R., Liber, J. M., Utens, E. M., & Treffers, P. D. (2011). Stepped care cognitive behavioural therapy for children with anxiety disorders: A new treatment approach. *Behavioural and Cognitive Psychotherapy, 39*(1), 55–75. doi:10.1017/s1352465810000500

Weisz, J. R., Chorpita, B. F., Frye, A., Ng, M. Y., Lau, N., Bearman, S. K., Ugueto, A. M., Langer, D. A., Hoagwood, K. E., and the Research Network on Youth Mental Health. (2011). Youth top problems: Using idiographic, consumer-guided assessment to identify treatment needs and to track change during psychotherapy. *Journal of Consulting and Clinical Psychology, 79*(3), 369–380. doi:10.1037/a0023307

World Health Organization. (2010). *Telemedicine: Opportunities and developments in member states. Report on the second global survey on eHealth.* World Health Organization Press.

11

Community Mental Health Delivery

ASHLEY M. SHAW, RENEE L. BROWN, VANESA A. MORA
RINGLE, AND VANESSA E. COBHAM ■

OVERVIEW OF COMMUNITY MENTAL HEALTH SETTINGS

Over the past five years, the Unified Protocol for Transdiagnostic Treatment of Emotional Disorders in Adolescents (UP-A) has been increasingly applied in community mental health settings across the United States and Australia. In the United States, it has been implemented in community mental health centers (CMHCs) in various states (e.g., Florida, Connecticut, and Texas). CMHCs were first established through federal funding in 1963 to increase availability of mental health services to all individuals in need (across socioeconomic status, race, and ethnicity) and to establish and coordinate mental health services that match the needs of specific communities (Dowell & Ciarlo, 1983). Thus, CMHCs are behavioral health clinics located within the communities or neighborhoods they serve and frequently serve low-income families (Dowell & Ciarlo, 1983). Services are paid for with insurance, such as Medicaid. In certain modern CMHCs, clinicians may offer home- and school-based services to reduce barriers to accessing care. Additionally, although CMHCs began as a government initiative, modern CMHCs may be for-profit or not-for-profit, publicly funded organizations. A large proportion of clinicians working at these agencies have their master's degrees, such as licensed mental health counselors licensed clinical social workers , and marriage and family counselors. CMHCs differ in their criteria for admission and available services, although many offer individual and family therapy, case management, and medication management.

The Australian counterparts of CMHCs are Child and Adolescent Mental Health Services. In Queensland, where the UP-A has been implemented, these services are known as Child and Youth Mental Health Services (CYMHS). The largest CYMHS in Queensland comprises hospital- and community-based teams and services (e.g., community outpatient clinics, alcohol and drug treatment services, e-mental health, inpatient family therapy, extended hours services, consultation liaison services, and specialist teams). These services cater to complex, severe presentations of youth up to age 18. Unlike in the United States, the Australian public health system does not require clients to have health insurance, and CYMHS are free of charge.

Upon presentation to the CYMHS, the youth's severity is assessed, which determines eligibility for outpatient or inpatient services. Eligibility for services is also based on whether the child could alternatively access private services and whether their presentation is appropriate for service within the community clinic or requires referral to specialized care within the larger service (e.g., an eating disorder clinic). Eligibility is determined collaboratively by the community clinic's team of mental health practitioners. For youth who are determined to be eligible, outpatient appointments occur on a weekly or fortnightly basis. The youth is assigned a principal service provider who provides individual and/or family therapy and parent sessions if appropriate. Additionally, the youth may participate in group therapy, medication management with the psychiatrist, and other services within CYMHS.

Community practice settings (CMHCs and CYMHS) present some challenges for implementing the UP-A because they differ from the provider and client populations in which the UP-A was developed and initially tested. In terms of unique provider characteristics, in initial UP-A trials the clinicians were largely doctoral students or postdoctoral fellows in clinical psychology (Ehrenreich-May et al., 2017), but community mental health clinicians come from a range of disciplines. For example, CMHC and CYMHS clinicians may have been trained through social work, counseling, psychology, clinical nursing, psychiatry, occupational therapy, or speech pathology. Due to the variety of training received across these disciplines, clinicians have variable levels of familiarity with cognitive-behavioral therapy (CBT). Relatedly, clinicians may hold different theoretical orientations (e.g., family systems or client-centered). Further, clinicians in community settings typically hold full, large caseloads and have difficulty finding time to immerse themselves in a new intervention in terms of training, supervision, and session planning. Additionally, to our knowledge, none of the community practices in these trials offered their employees incentives for learning a new evidence-based treatment or doing it with fidelity. Particularly at CMHCs where home- and school-based services are offered, CMHC clinicians have quite hectic schedules, driving from one location to another throughout the day. The combination of less familiarity with CBT and a lack of time to engage in comprehensive training presents barriers for clinicians in community settings to adopt an evidence-based, manualized treatment like the UP-A (Cobham et al., 2018).

In terms of the client population, clients in these settings have complex and severe presentations, which differ from those seen in typical research-based settings. For example, in the Australian CYMHS, the majority of youth experience suicidal ideation, self-harm, and/or a history of suicide attempt(s). Compared to initial UP-A trials (e.g., Ehrenreich-May et al., 2017), across both U.S. and Australian community settings, clients present more often with comorbid depression, a history of interpersonal trauma, family conflict, and multiple comorbidities.

Clients treated in U.S. CMHCs are also demographically different from original UP-A samples, including more youth from low-income and African American backgrounds. Overall, clients seen in community settings tend to face substantially more treatment barriers than those typically seen in university clinics (Weisz et al., 2013, 2015).

ADAPTATIONS TO UP-A IN COMMUNITY MENTAL HEALTH SETTINGS

In the context of ongoing and completed UP-A trials in the CYMHS and CMHC settings conducted by Cobham, Ehrenreich-May, and collaborators, clinicians have made several adaptations to UP-A delivery to meet their particular clients' needs. These adaptations were made to the UP-A format, content, and materials.

Format

In the CYMHS, clients commonly dropped out of treatment earlier than is typical in research settings, so a portion of youth in the community trial received an abbreviated treatment. Clients in the CYMHS are discharged at age 18, so engaged 17-year-olds were taken through specific UP-A modules, selected based on their presentation. This treatment format was approached with the knowledge that the time the young person could engage in therapy was limited and ensured that the most relevant content was delivered to the youth while they were enrolled in therapy. Across both U.S. and Australian trials, such an approach was also indicated for any youth whose treatment course was limited due to a practical and foreseeable constraint (e.g., anticipated lack of insurance or plans to relocate outside of the catchment area). An example of an accelerated UP-A approach used by a CYMHS clinician for an engaged 17-year-old with social anxiety is included in Box 11.1. In this example, the sequencing of the UP-A modules was altered for increased efficiency and personalization. Indeed, in CYMHS, where treatment engagement was variable and often limited, clinicians often chose to prioritize modules that they perceived were most relevant for the client's presentation. Modules were also prioritized for specific presentations, such as Module 7 for school refusal.

Another common scenario in the CYMHS trial was that clients were engaged in the service for an extended period of time, but UP-A delivery was derailed by the client's complexities. In the CYMHS trial, the number of sessions with such clients may have exceeded 30, but many of these sessions were focused on risk management or a recent crisis event. In these scenarios, reviewing UP-A content was often required after addressing crises during previous sessions. Although this further delayed introducing new concepts, clinicians found it necessary to refresh the adolescent on the knowledge gained from previous sessions. When client risk

Box 11.1

SAMPLE THERAPIST MODULE OUTLINE

UP-A Module 1: Building and Keeping Motivation (1 or 2 sessions)

Materials Needed for This Module
- Worksheet 1.1, "Defining the Main Problems"
- Worksheet 1.2, "Weighing My Options"
- Appendix 1.2, "Defining the Main Problems—Parent Form"
- Appendix 1.3, "Weekly Top Problems Tracking Form"

Goal 1—Orient Adolescent and Family to the UP-A (necessary)
- Overview of the UP-A
  - Explain that the UP-A aims to help teens manage strong or intense emotions in more helpful ways.
  - Explain a general timeline for treatment.
  - Emphasize the importance of home learning assignments.
- Provide the parent with Worksheet 1.1, "Defining the Main Problems— Parent Form" to complete.
- Clarify level of parent involvement desired by the adolescent.

Goal 2—Establish Top Problems and SMART Goals (necessary)
- Identify the adolescent's three Top Problems using Worksheet 1.1.
- Use Appendix 1.3, "Weekly Top Problems Tracking Form," to have the adolescent rate the severity of their Top Problems today.
- Note: Suicidal ideation and/or self-harm behaviors should be added to this list of Top Problems even if the adolescent does not think they are a problem. Clinician can add these, emphasizing our concern for client safety and well-being.
- Generate the SMART goals, using the second half of Worksheet 1.1.

Goal 3—Further Address Adolescent Motivation for Treatment (optional)
- Look at the SMART goals and work with the adolescent to identify actionable "baby steps" that might be helpful in achieving these goals.
- Use strategies for evoking change talk (see the therapist guide)—for example, explore the pros and cons of change; look forward to the future to figure out whether current behaviors are helping your adolescent to achieve what they want from life.
- Do the "Decisional Balance" exercise (Worksheet 1.2, "Weighing My Options") and ideally secure commitment to continuing with therapy (for the next few sessions at minimum) to see if the benefits can outweigh the disadvantages.

Goal 4—Parent Motivational Enhancement (optional)
- Review and assess the appropriateness of the parent's Top Problem list.
- Assess the parent's motivation to participate in their adolescent's treatment, normalizing barriers for parental involvement and identifying specific barriers for this parent that might interfere with their ability to participate.
- Use motivational enhancement strategies to try to engage a parent whose motivation is low.

Home Learning
- Nothing defined for this module—however, there may be things you want either your adolescent or their parent to do (e.g., parent to think about potential barriers to their involvement in treatment).

---

and crises dominated treatment, clinicians were encouraged by their supervisor to weave UP-A content into the session where appropriate. This called for using specific UP-A tools out of their traditional sequence. For example, the "Tracking the Before, During, and After" and "Problem Solving" forms represented useful tools across the U.S. and Australian trials to explore reactions to and solutions for a given crisis the young person was experiencing. Where this was not appropriate, the UP-A was "paused" and the clinician returned to it when the client's immediate risk had been managed.

Content

Several specific adaptations to UP-A psychoeducation have occurred in the ongoing CYMHS trial. For example, several older adolescents expressed interest in the biological basis of their symptoms. In response, clinicians expanded upon emotion education with the use of evolutionary metaphors introduced at the beginning of Goal 2 in Module 2 and Goal 1 in Module 4. Specifically, one clinician reflected upon the usefulness of anxiety as a protective mechanism necessary for survival for cavemen because it served to protect them against predators and other dangers inherent in the prehistoric environment. They shared with the adolescent:

Anxiety is an important response to what's happening in our environment, and we can understand this in terms of our ancestors. When humans lived in caves, they faced all different life-threatening situations. If a saber-toothed tiger was seen, we can imagine that this would have caused feelings of anxiety. These feelings alerted the caveman that they needed to escape the threat. If the caveman didn't feel anxiety and felt relaxed with predators around, we can imagine they would not have survived very long. The feelings of anxiety that the caveman experienced may not have differed much to how we respond when we are faced with a threatening situation; it's just that our threats are quite different, as the environment for humans has changed.

Expansion of the psychoeducation in the CYMHS trial has also included additional information about the threat response following traumatic experiences, since many young clients in CYMHS settings had experienced interpersonal trauma. Clinicians may benefit from referring to other manualized interventions targeted to youth who have experienced trauma (e.g., trauma-focused cognitive-behavioral therapy; Cohen & Mannarino, 2017) for a more formal discussion of specific psychoeducation about the trauma response.

Materials

One adaptation to UP-A materials in community settings included flexibility about the use of worksheets. School refusal, both in terms of attendance and work completion, is a common presenting problem in community settings. Youth with school refusal recruited into these trials were often resistant to engaging with workbooks and worksheets, as these materials reminded them of school. In such scenarios, community clinicians engaged in a variety of approaches to suit the preference of the young person. For example, clinicians either (1) talked through the UP-A content without using the workbook or engaging with any of the worksheets or forms, (2) transcribed the worksheet content to a whiteboard with the young person, for interactive completion, or (3) incorporated the adolescent's mobile device for worksheet completion. Some youth who did not want to use worksheets or take notes during session were still open to taking pictures of key worksheets (e.g., the "Detective Questions"), writing out the "Tracking the Before, During, and After" form in the notes section of their phone, or tracking their emotions on an app (e.g., Daylio).

Across both trials, module outlines were created for quick reference in session to facilitate clinicians' implementation of the UP-A with recruited participants. The module outlines consisted of up to a few short pages dedicated to each module. The module outlines used in the CYMHS trial consisted of the following information:

- A list of the worksheets and forms that the clinician would need for that module;
- A summary of the module goals, and which goals were optional;
- Within each goal, the main content to be covered.

Box 11.1 shows a one-page example of a Module 1 outline used in CYMHS settings. Of note is the addition of suicidal ideation and/or self-harm as a mandatory Top Problem when present in the young person, as this presentation was common in the CYMHS setting.

ONGOING RESEARCH ON UP-A IMPLEMENTATION IN COMMUNITY MENTAL HEALTH SETTINGS

The largest U.S. trial examining the effectiveness of the UP-A in CMHCs is the Community Study of Outcome Monitoring for Emotional Disorders in Teens (COMET; Jensen-Doss et al., 2018), which recently completed data collection. Inclusion criteria for this trial were (1) being age 12 to 18, (2) having clinically significant symptoms of an anxiety, obsessive-compulsive, or depressive disorder, (3) being deemed appropriate for outpatient services by the CMHC, (4) living with a guardian who was willing to attend sessions, and (5) being able to speak and read in English or Spanish. Youth were excluded if they were receiving another psychosocial intervention (excluding case management or medication management), if they exhibited suicidal behavior that was too severe for outpatient treatment, or if their presentation was contraindicated for UP-A (e.g., low IQ or primary substance use problem). Participants were identified after calling the CMHC and being screened for eligibility by the study team. Compared to the initial UP-A efficacy trials, the COMET trial had several adaptations. For example, some clinicians saw clients in their home or school rather than in the office. Additionally, some CMHCs approved weekly two-hour sessions for clients whose presentation was particularly severe. In these scenarios, clinicians generally split the session in half, meeting with the adolescent for the first half and reviewing adolescent content and Module P material with the parent in the second hour of the session. A major difference from previous UP-A trials, due to study design (for more details see Jensen-Doss et al., 2018), was that all clinicians also administered the Youth Outcome Questionnaire (YOQ; Burlingame et al., 2005) each session to monitor client outcomes, reviewed graphical YOQ feedback, and provided feedback to families based on the results of the YOQ. Another difference from previous trials was that there was no maximum number of UP-A sessions allowed; thus, cases could be seen beyond the 21-session maximum used in the initial open trial (Ehrenreich-May et al., 2017).

In the Australian community trial of the UP-A conducted in CYMHS community settings, inclusion criteria were that clients (1) were 12 to 18 years old, (2) presented with a primary anxiety and/or depressive disorder, and (3) were starting a new CYMHS service episode. Clients were included in the trial if they presented with comorbidity or with suicidal ideation and/or self-harm and if they had been a previous client of the service, with the last service episode occurring greater than one year prior. Clients were excluded from the trial only if individual therapy was not engaged in (e.g., if suicidality was such that case management dominated the services utilized) or if they were unable to engage with cognitively based material (i.e., due to low IQ). Participants were identified and recruited into the trial by community CYMHS clinicians. The major modification from traditional UP-A in the CYMHS trial was that, when it was acceptable for both the youth and the caregiver(s), the caregiver(s) were invited to sit in for most of each session with the youth, with the end of the session spent with the youth only. This adaptation followed feedback from community CYMHS clinicians, who felt that caregivers would themselves benefit from the content delivered to youth from the UP-A.

EXAMPLE OF A COMMUNITY MENTAL HEALTH CLINICIAN'S IMPLEMENTATION OF THE UP-A

Next, we will present an illustrative case example of a community clinician as they moved through various stages of comfort with the UP-A. "Sarah"[1] was a 29-year-old social worker who had been working in CYMHS for approximately 18 months when the UP-A effectiveness trial commenced. She had previously worked in the public adult mental health system. Since beginning in CYMHS, Sarah had been particularly proactive in seeking out professional development opportunities, in part because she had felt quite anxious about working with children, adolescents, and families. Sarah described her primary theoretical orientation as family therapy. At the beginning of her clinic's involvement in the trial, Sarah described herself as a "hesitant but willing" participant clinician—with the hesitance being due to her belief that evidence-based manualized interventions were unlikely to be effective or relevant for the complex CYMHS population. Sarah noted that she was grateful for the opportunity to participate in the two-day UP-A training and to receive fortnightly UP-A supervision, as she had not been formally trained in or used CBT previously. Sarah volunteered to be the "clinic champion" for her team, attended the majority of supervisions offered, and consistently encouraged her colleagues to recruit families to the trial.

Sarah had not previously been involved in or exposed to a research project and initially was concerned about deviating in any way from the UP-A therapist guide. For example, in discussing her first session with her first UP-A case in supervision, Sarah expressed her worry that in using a goal-setting tool (which was not part of the UP-A) to help the adolescent generate Top Problems and SMART goals, she had compromised the case in terms of the effectiveness trial and the research protocol. Importantly, this uncertainty about UP-A fidelity was a common and recurring theme for clinicians as they worked through the UP-A with their initial clients. Once Sarah understood that it was acceptable to not follow the therapist guide to the letter, and as her familiarity with the content increased, Sarah became highly skilled at weaving key content from different modules across sessions (as opposed to moving in a linear fashion through the therapist guide). This meant that the content being presented was always relevant to client concerns raised in that session, whether this was responding to an adolescent's recount of a romantic/friendship conflict or assessing and managing crisis situations. Sarah commented, "I found it really tough at the start [because] I felt like . . . I had to stay within the module. But . . . as supervision's gone on [I realized it was OK to] focus

1. The name and other identifying information for this therapist has been changed to maintain anonymity.

on [the overarching] goals. So you might cover a goal from one module and a goal from another module [in one session] . . . to get some traction [with the client] or to address the concern that a young person comes with [on that day]."

Over the course of more than 10 clients enrolled in the effectiveness trial, Sarah made two setting-specific adaptations to the UP-A. First, Sarah moved Module 7 content (situational emotional exposure) forward so that it was covered earlier (typically after or in parallel with Module 2 content). This adaptation was made by most clinicians in our trial. The clients for whom Sarah made this adaptation were adolescents who were not attending school. Sarah felt that it was important to begin working on the emotional behavior of avoidance (often one of the client's Top Problems) as early as possible. Bringing this content in earlier meant that clients (and caregivers) felt that one of their most pressing problems was being worked on from an early point in therapy. It also often had the consequence of providing clients with some early experiences of success, which was helpful in terms of both client motivation and the therapeutic relationship. Second, Sarah covered the present-moment awareness content of Module 6 ahead of the cognitive content of Module 5. Sarah made this adaptation in two cases where the adolescent clients had a high level of perfectionism. For instance, in the first case where this came up, Sarah had initially thought that the 17-year-old adolescent (a previously high academic achiever who had become "paralyzed" by his perfectionism and anxiety such that he was no longer willing to even attempt any schoolwork) would engage with and respond well to the Module 5 content. However, once she started this module with her client, Sarah observed that he appeared to view his engagement in different thinking traps as further evidence of his own inadequacy. After discussion in supervision, Sarah talked to her client about taking a different direction. The present-moment awareness content was experienced as extremely helpful by the adolescent and set the scene for beginning Module 5 afresh.

Sarah became one of our most experienced and effective UP-A clinicians. She now mentors peers around utilizing the UP-A and has been a valuable member of the supervision group, often coming up with creative ideas about how to make use of UP-A content in her peers' cases. Sarah's treatment adherence has been excellent, and she views the UP-A training, supervision, and implementation as critical to her professional development. Sarah found that, due to her experience with the UP-A and the implementation support put in place around it in the effectiveness trial, her views about the usefulness of a manualized intervention with a CYMHS population had changed markedly. In her own words:

> Before I started using the UP-A I would have said it had a limited sort of role [with CYMHS clients] . . . typically our consumer population's quite chaotic, and I would have thought a tailored approach would be a lot more suitable . . . But since doing UP-A I've [come] to consider more consumers eligible to . . . use that, and [find] it effective. I've seen some good results so far with the UP-A; and it's helpful [to me]—[to have] something that's manualized but flexible.

TROUBLESHOOTING BARRIERS TO IMPLEMENTING
THE UP-A IN COMMUNITY SETTINGS

We recounted the experience of a community clinician, Sarah, in which she noted initially having difficulty knowing how closely to maintain fidelity to the UP-A. Concern about UP-A fidelity is one of various UP-A implementation barriers that community clinicians may encounter. In this section we outline common intervention-, clinician-, and client-level barriers to UP-A implementation in community settings based on anecdotal data and data collected via semistructured interviews with community clinicians (after their participation in the COMET study; Jensen-Doss et al., 2018). We also suggest ways to overcome these barriers.

Intervention Barriers

Intervention-level barriers refer to UP-A characteristics (i.e., the written materials and supplemental materials) that hinder its usage by clinicians working in community settings. For example, the challenge of balancing fidelity to a manualized intervention with the flexibility needed in community settings is common to many manualized treatment approaches (Ringle et al., 2015). Notably, given that the UP-A is a transdiagnostic, modular treatment, various developmental iterations of the Unified Protocols are often highlighted by researchers for their flexible nature (see McHugh et al., 2009). Nevertheless, it appears that the message of the UP-A as a flexible, modular approach is not at the forefront of clinicians' minds, as they still report feeling troubled that they may be deviating from the manual in potentially detrimental ways. To overcome this barrier, the flexibility and adaptability of the UP-A must be stressed throughout training, supervision, and consultation. As knowledge grew about this intervention barrier throughout the COMET trial, flexibility was emphasized more in consultation during the latter half of the trial, particularly around giving explicit recommendations to do modules out of order, to include material from multiple modules in one session, and to flexibly use UP-A material to address a crisis of the week. Supervisors and consultants leading future trainings should repetitively emphasize the UP-A's flexibility (e.g., with vignettes of what it would look like to veer off course) and concretely identify what types of deviations from the UP-A would be unhelpful or detrimental. It may also be helpful for the next edition of the UP-A therapist guide to highlight opportunities for flexibility even more.

Another intervention-related barrier reported by community clinicians included the length and comprehensiveness of the UP-A therapist guide. To address this barrier, both effectiveness trials used module summaries or "cheat sheets" (see Box 11.1) to facilitate its implementation in CMHCs. Many community therapists reported that balancing learning a new treatment approach with existing work demands (e.g., heavy caseloads, travel to and from sessions) was difficult, and having these brief outlines simplified their use of UP-A content/ strategies and need to remember many details. Additionally, many community therapists suggested that reading the adolescent workbook was a more straightforward, time-efficient approach to prepare for sessions than reviewing the corresponding chapter of the therapist guide.

Many clinicians also indicated that it would be helpful to have the UP-A therapist guide, parent handouts, and the adolescent workbook available in languages other than English. For example, one clinician stated that the UP-A "should have . . . more work in Spanish . . . I'm thinking about necessity and diversity in [the community in which I work] . . . it would be nice to have it in another language." Notably, some COMET clinicians did use unpublished UP-A materials that were available in Spanish. Fortunately, final versions of the UP-A materials are now published in several languages, including Spanish.

Clinician Barriers

The Consolidated Framework for Implementation Research (Damschroder et al., 2009) is a theory that describes factors that impact the implementation of an intervention and includes the characteristics of individuals involved—such as the clinicians—as well as the process of implementation. Clinician-level barriers refer to individual clinician factors, in the context of organizational limitations, that hamper UP-A implementation. Relatedly, time constraints and large caseloads in CMHCs emerged as implementation obstacles for community UP-A clinicians, and these have been noted as common clinician barriers to implementing evidence-based treatments in previous effectiveness trials (e.g., Becker-Haimes et al., 2017). Since large caseloads will often be the case for community clinicians, we hope to provide some recommendations for easing the process of learning and adopting a new practice such as the UP-A. For example, in our UP-A community trials, time constraints were partially addressed through the module summaries, and time in consultation was spent engaging in brief but active learning approaches (e.g., practicing through role plays). Additionally, clinicians in training should feel comfortable engaging in supervision or consultation on the UP-A as their circumstances allow. For example, many of our clinicians in the COMET study called in to receive consultation while driving. Naturally, time allocations and caseloads are determined at the organizational level; thus, facilitating the implementation of the UP-A may also require organizational-level strategies (e.g., increasing educational and leadership support in implementing interventions; Powell et al., 2017).

Another barrier for community clinicians was lacking access to printers and copy machines to provide UP-A handouts to clients and families, particularly if they were doing home visits and traveling between appointments. To troubleshoot this obstacle, the clinician could do one or more of the following: (1) use the freely available UP-A handouts in fillable PDF format from the Oxford University Press on their laptop or (2) create a binder of the freely available UP-A handouts with clear protective coversheets so that they can write and rewrite on the handouts across clients and sessions with a dry erase marker.

Community clinicians also noted attitudes and beliefs that may have hindered their usage of the UP-A. For example, one U.S. clinician commented, "I think [the UP-A] is very different from, or somewhat different . . . from, the way that we're trained and we practice here, and I am just obviously much more inclined to the way we practice than the UP-A." This comment suggests that learning the UP-A may not have been as appealing as the interventions they were already using, which may have led the integration of this new treatment into their practice to be viewed as a stressor rather than an opportunity, when faced with heavy caseload demands. Another barrier was completing enough UP-A cases to feel competent. Some clinicians felt that completing one UP-A case was insufficient to feel competent in UP-A delivery and that delivering the UP-A became easier with more practice. In this regard, some therapists suggested that short videos demonstrating the delivery of UP-A techniques might be helpful. Indeed, the treatment developers are working on developing additional brief videos on UP-A techniques to facilitate continued learning after the initial training.

Client Barriers

Client-level barriers refer to adolescent or parent characteristics that unintentionally interfere with UP-A implementation. Client-level barriers associated with UP-A implementation in community settings parallel barriers previously documented in the literature (Ringle et al., 2015), including youth experiencing comorbid posttraumatic stress disorder (PTSD), poverty, and family instability. Given its transdiagnostic nature focused on an array of emotional disorders, the UP-A may be able to address traumatic stress disorders in adolescents. However, therapists in the COMET trial reported that trauma histories and PTSD diagnoses made it more challenging to implement the UP-A, given the complexity of these client presentations. Indeed, one of these clinicians noted, "Being in a community mental health center . . . the population we work with typically has a lot of needs because they're impoverished, and have a high amount of trauma in their history." In terms of treating clients in the context of poverty and family instability, UP-A therapists in community settings should be informed of culturally sensitive strategies for engaging traditionally underserved populations (i.e., people with economic, cultural, or linguistic barriers to health care) in the face of multiple stressors (U.S. Department of Health and Human Services, 2001). One example includes matching the cultural background of the therapist and the client (Kazak et al., 2010; Park et al., 2020). Most importantly, clients should be matched with a therapist fluent in their primary language.

We also would like to note unique challenges to involving caregivers in UP-A treatment in community settings. Given that this is a treatment for adolescents, parents sometimes expect to be involved only minimally or not at all, which poses a barrier for clinicians trying to adhere to UP-A treatment recommendations for level of parent involvement. Given this barrier, community therapists would do well to collaboratively set expectations for treatment involvement with parents at the initial sessions. Additionally, community therapists may be providing the UP-A in school settings, thus limiting their ability to involve parents. Under these circumstances, therapists should be encouraged to make their best efforts to creatively incorporate parents. For clinicians providing UP-A in the school setting or other situations when the primary caregiver cannot be present at each session, we would recommend trying to incorporate parents in one or more of the following ways. Clinicians could send UP-A parent handouts home with the child so the parent is aware of the content covered, initiate a five- to 10-minute weekly call with the parent to inform them of key points of the session and the assigned home learning, and/or try to have at least one session per month that the parent can attend.

Other times, parents were very involved in their adolescent's treatment, but conflict between the parent and child posed a barrier to the traditional UP-A format. If the material in Module P is insufficient for troubleshooting emotional parenting behaviors (e.g., inconsistency or criticism), we recommend providing parents with the UP-C parent workbook, which contains a fuller discussion of addressing emotional parenting behaviors. In scenarios when parental criticism during session affects the adolescent's engagement or motivation, we would recommend keeping meetings with the adolescent and parent separate to the extent possible until both the adolescent and parent have developed coping strategies, which can be later rehearsed during exposure. When conducting exposures around high-distress conversation topics between parents and adolescents, we recommend preparing both the parent and the adolescent (in separate check-ins) with a behavioral goal to engage in opposite actions and/or opposite parenting behaviors. All parties should be aware that the goal of the exposure is not to resolve the conflict but to practice using opposite actions and opposite parenting behaviors when distress is high between parent and child.

Finally, there were also logistical client barriers that shortened the ideal length of treatment. For example, in the United States, many families had to end treatment prematurely due to a lapse in insurance coverage. To troubleshoot this barrier, we have started exploring brief, streamlined versions of the UP-A (e.g., Handout 1 and Chapter 10), which take into account which core skills might be most impactful for the given adolescent. However, if insurance coverage ended abruptly, with less notice, we would recommend at least having a termination session (i.e., Module 8) to review skills learned so far, develop a plan to help the adolescent cope with emotional triggers during the lapse of therapy, and continued goal setting. Another logistical barrier in community settings can be unstable housing. In the COMET study, many children moved between two caregivers' homes or relocated during treatment. With the growing use and acceptance of telehealth across CMHCs during the COVID-19 pandemic, hopefully relocation is no longer a barrier, as providers could finish the course of the UP-A via telehealth. See Chapter 10 for more details on delivering UP-A via telehealth.

SUMMARY

The UP-A has been applied in community mental health settings to diverse adolescents by community clinicians across the United States and Australia. We have summarized adaptations that were commonly used by community clinicians, such as abbreviating the UP-A and utilizing module summaries. We also described the case of Sarah, a community mental health clinician in CYMHS, who initially worried about veering too far from UP-A content and order but later was able to flexibly apply and re-order UP-A content to best suit her client. Finally, we summarized intervention-level, clinician-level, and client-level barriers for implementing the UP-A in community settings and provided recommendations for clinicians, supervisors, and consultants about how to troubleshoot these barriers. Overall, the UP-A was created as a modular, transdiagnostic intervention to allow flexible application across a range of settings, and we hope community clinicians, supervisors, and agencies consider applying this intervention flexibly to their unique client population.

Tip Sheet for Implementing the UP-A in Community Mental Health Settings

Helpful UP-A Adaptations in Community Settings

- ✓ If you need to do an abbreviated treatment because the treatment course is shortened by logistical barriers, think about which key skills will be most important for that client. It's acceptable to skip modules and go out of order for increased personalization and efficiency.
- ✓ You may need to integrate additional psychoeducation (e.g., on trauma reactions) depending on the client's diagnostic presentation.
- ✓ Try using "cheat sheets" or one- or two-page outlines that summarize the key content you'll want to cover in each module.
- ✓ Introduce Module 7 earlier, particularly if school refusal is present.
- ✓ Depending on the relationship between parent and child (i.e., low conflict), it may be helpful to have the parent present for the majority of sessions, particularly if the parent also experiences psychological symptoms and could benefit from using the skills as well.
- ✓ It is always helpful to have the "Tracking the Before, During, and After" and "Problem Solving" worksheets on hand, as they can be helpful in applying a UP-A concept to a new crisis in the client's life.
- ✓ If you have been approved for two-hour weekly sessions with a severe client, consider meeting with the adolescent for the first hour and reviewing child content and Module P material with the parent in second hour of the session.

Barriers and Solutions

BARRIER	SOLUTION
Are you worried about doing UP-A perfectly, exactly as the therapist guide outlines?	Remember that the UP-A is flexible. Consult with UP-A experts/trainers about using the UP-A flexibly.
Do you have a large caseload and little time to review all of the UP-A materials?	Prioritize reviewing the UP-A workbook; use "cheat sheets."
Are you concerned that the UP-A won't apply to your diverse clients from underserved backgrounds?	Keep doing the culturally sensitive care you have been trained in while teaching your client UP-A skills. Adapt the UP-A as necessary.
Did you devote one or more sessions to risk management or a crisis?	If appropriate, try to weave UP-A material into handling the crisis. It's acceptable and indicated to take time to review UP-A material at the next session.

Is your client resistant to using worksheets?

Try a whiteboard or have them use their mobile phone.

Are you unable to carry all of your UP-A materials from session to session or have limited access to extra copies of the workbook or a printer?

Use the freely available handouts from the Oxford University Press or create a binder of handouts with protective, reusable coversheets.

Do you see your client at school and wonder how to incorporate parents?

Send the parent handouts, do a brief weekly call, or encourage their presence in at least one session per month.

Situations Where UP-A Would Not Be Appropriate to Use in a Community Setting

- When PTSD is primary and trauma-focused CBT is available at the clinic
- When a client is chronically suicidal and requires a higher level of care

ACKNOWLEDGMENT

Funding for some of the research presented in this chapter was provided by the Children's Hospital Foundation, Queensland, Australia.

REFERENCES

Becker-Haimes, E. M., Okamura, K. H., Wolk, C. B., Rubin, R., Evans, A. C., & Beidas, R. S. (2017). Predictors of clinician use of exposure therapy in community mental health settings. *Journal of Anxiety Disorders, 49*, 88–94. doi:10.1016/j.janxdis.2017.04.002

Burlingame, G., Cox, J., Wells, G., Latkowski, M., Justice, D., Carter, C., & Lambert, M. (2005). *The administration and scoring manual of the Youth Outcome Questionnaire.* OQ Measures.

Cobham, V. E., Brown, R., Stathis, S., & Ehrenreich-May, J. (2018). *Attitudes towards evidence-based treatments: A qualitative study of community child and youth mental health clinicians.* Paper presented at the European Association of Behavioural and Cognitive Therapies, Sofia, Bulgaria.

Cohen, J. A., Mannarino, A. P., & Deblinger, E. (2017). *Treating trauma and traumatic grief in children and adolescents* (2nd ed.). Guilford Press.

Damschroder, L. J., Aron, D. C., Keith, R. E., Kirsh, S. R., Alexander, J. A., & Lowery, J. C. (2009). Fostering implementation of health services research findings into practice: A consolidated framework for advancing implementation science. *Implementation Science, 4*(1), 50. doi:10.1186/1748-5908-4-50

Dowell, D. A., & Ciarlo, J. A. (1983). Overview of the Community Mental Health Centers Program from an evaluation perspective. *Community Mental Health Journal, 19*(2), 95–128. doi:10.1007/bf00877603

Ehrenreich-May, J., Rosenfield, D., Queen, A. H., Kennedy, S. M., Remmes, C. S., & Barlow, D. H. (2017). An initial waitlist-controlled trial of the unified protocol for the treatment of emotional disorders in adolescents. *Journal of Anxiety Disorders, 46*, 46–55. doi:10.1016/j.janxdis.2016.10.006

Jensen-Doss, A., Ehrenreich-May, J., Nanda, M. M., Maxwell, C. A., LoCurto, J., Shaw, A. M., Souer, H., Rosenfield, D., & Ginsburg, G. S. (2018). Community Study of Outcome Monitoring for Emotional Disorders in Teens (COMET): A comparative effectiveness trial of a transdiagnostic treatment and a measurement feedback system. *Contemporary Clinical Trials, 74*, 18–24. doi:10.1016/j.cct.2018.09.011

Kazak, A. E., Hoagwood, K., Weisz, J. R., Hood, K., Kratochwill, T. R., Vargas, L. A., & Banez, G. A. (2010). A meta-systems approach to evidence-based practice for children and adolescents. *American Psychologist, 65*(2), 85.

McHugh, R. K., Murray, H. W., & Barlow, D. H. (2009). Balancing fidelity and adaptation in the dissemination of empirically-supported treatments: The promise of transdiagnostic interventions. *Behaviour Research and Therapy, 47*(11), 946–953. doi:10.1016/j.brat.2009.07.005

Park, A. L., Boustani, M. M., Saifan, D., Gellatly, R., Letamendi, A., Stanick, C., Regan, J., Perez, G., Manners, D., Reding, M. E. J., & Chorpita, B. F. (2020). Community mental health professionals' perceptions about engaging underserved populations. *Administration and Policy in Mental Health, 47*(3), 366–379.

Powell, B. J., Mandell, D. S., Hadley, T. R., Rubin, R. M., Evans, A. C., Hurford, M. O., & Beidas, R. S. (2017). Are general and strategic measures of organizational context and leadership associated with knowledge and attitudes toward evidence-based practices in public behavioral health settings? A cross-sectional observational study. *Implementation Science, 2*(1), 64.

Ringle, V. A., Read, K. L., Edmunds, J. M., Brodman, D. M., Kendall, P. C., Barg, F., & Beidas, R. S. (2015). Barriers to and facilitators in the implementation of cognitive-behavioral therapy for youth anxiety in the community. *Psychiatric Services, 66*(9), 938–945.

U.S. Department of Health and Human Services. (2001). *Mental health: Culture, race, and ethnicity—A supplement to mental health: A report of the Surgeon General.*

Weisz, J. R., Krumholz, L. S., Santucci, L., Thomassin, K., & Ng, M. Y. (2015). Shrinking the gap between research and practice: Tailoring and testing youth psychotherapies in clinical care contexts. *Annual Review of Clinical Psychology, 11*(1), 139–163. doi:10.1146/annurev-clinpsy-032814-112820

Weisz, J. R., Ugueto, A. M., Cheron, D. M., & Herren, J. (2013). Evidence-based youth psychotherapy in the mental health ecosystem. *Journal of Clinical Child & Adolescent Psychology, 42*(2), 274–286. doi:10.1080/15374416.2013.764824

12

Culturally and Linguistically Sensitive Applications in Other Countries

HIROKO FUJISATO, NORIKO KATO, DOMINIQUE PHILLIPS, AND ESTEFANY SÁEZ-CLARKE ■

CULTURAL ADAPTATIONS IN EVIDENCE-BASED PRACTICE

When providing a psychological service using evidence-based practice, the service rendered should be suitable for the client's characteristics, culture, and preferences (American Psychological Association, 2006). Cultural adaptation, which maintains a balance between scientifically rigorous interventions and culturally effective practice, is defined as "the systematic modification of an evidence-based treatment (EBT) or intervention protocol to consider language, culture, and context in such a way that it is compatible with the client's cultural patterns, meanings, and values" (Bernal et al., 2009). In past meta-analyses designed to verify the effectiveness of cultural adaptation in psychotherapy, interventions provided to a specific cultural group were four times more effective than interventions provided to groups comprising clients with various cultural backgrounds. In addition, interventions conducted in clients' native language (if other than English) were twice as effective as interventions conducted in English (Griner & Smith, 2006), and culturally adapted psychotherapy has been reported to be more effective than unadapted psychotherapy (Benish et al., 2011).

Cognitive-behavioral therapy (CBT), such as the Unified Protocols for Transdiagnostic Treatment of Emotional Disorders in Children and Adolescents (UP-C/A), is an evidence-based psychotherapy that has mainly been developed and evaluated in Western cultures. However, the application of CBT in the context of other cultures has not been adequately studied. Recently, a shift toward the cultural adaptation of CBT has been proposed, on the basis of respecting and acting in accordance with the client's culture and employing an explanatory model that suits the client's needs and cultural values (Hays, 2009; Hinton & Patel, 2017). In this chapter, we introduce an adaptation of the UP-C/A within the context of Japanese culture, including a specific case study of a cultural and linguistic adaptation of the UP-C/A.

ADAPTING THE UP-C/A WITHIN THE CONTEXT OF JAPANESE CULTURE

When introducing the UP-C/A into a new cultural context, translating the treatment may be sufficient in some countries and regions, while others may require more systematic modification. In Japan, the UP-C was adapted using the following steps:

1. The original therapist guide and workbook were translated into Japanese.
2. The intervention was administered to one child and their mother using the translated texts.
3. Using the responses of the family as reference, five clinicians identified needed adaptations and prepared a revised version.
4. The intervention was administered in a group setting using the revised version.
5. Using the responses of the families as reference, three clinicians made minor adjustments to the expressions and other aspects of the therapist guide and workbook to finalize the adaptation.

The UP-A was adapted using the following steps:

1. The original therapist guide and workbook were translated into Japanese.
2. Four clinicians reviewed and modified them, referring to the modifications made in the UP-C and taking into consideration the target age range of the UP-A.
3. The intervention was administered to one adolescent and their parent using the revised versions.
4. Using the responses of the family as reference, two clinicians made minor adjustments to the expressions and other aspects of the therapist guide and workbook to finalize the adaptations.

In the following section, we specify the cultural and linguistic challenges that we encountered while preparing the Japanese UP-C/A and describe ways in which such issues were resolved. The UP-C intervention targets children and required significant modifications to make it a more enjoyable and accessible program. Like the UP for adults, however, the UP-A did not require notable modifications.

Adapting Program Names

In Japan, the stigma attached to mental disorders is still robust (Ando et al., 2013; Masuda et al., 2009; Yoshioka et al., 2014). Therefore, in Japanese settings, if the titles of intervention manuals contain words such as "emotional disorders" or "treatment," families in need of services often find it quite difficult to accept or engage with the intervention. Thus, instead of using a direct Japanese translation of the treatment title (i.e., "Unified Protocol for Transdiagnostic Treatment of Emotional Disorders"), the Japanese workbooks and therapist guides were titled "Emotion Detectives Program for Children" and "Program to Use Emotions as an Ally for Teenagers," to represent the UP-C and UP-A respectively. We noted, however, that the revised titles had the potential to confuse researchers and clinicians seeking to use the UP-C/A adaptations, as the target and content of the treatments were ambiguous. To resolve this issue, we incorporated the manuals into a series entitled the "Unified Protocols of Cognitive-Behavioral Therapy to Manage Emotions Skillfully" in hopes of fostering the acceptability of the programs to potential clients and therapists.

Adapting CLUES Skill Names

Within the UP-C, there are five core emotion management skills, represented by the acronym "CLUES," used to introduce the idea that throughout treatment, children are gathering clues to solve their own emotional mysteries. While this mnemonic is accessible to English-speaking children, Japanese children found the acronym unfamiliar and difficult to understand. As a result, the five skill names used in the original version of UP-C required modification.

An acronym such as "CLUES" could have been used in Japanese as well; however, it was extremely difficult to fulfill all the required conditions (i.e., using skill names easily understood by Japanese children that formed a memorable acronym, while still corresponding to each skill that "CLUES" represents). Thus, in the Japanese version, new names for the five "Emotion Detective Skills" were created: "Crime Scene Investigation," "Culprit Identification," "Evidence Collection and Strategy Planning," "Confrontation," and "Master Detective," with each skill corresponding to the C, L, U, E, and S skills, respectively. These skill names were easily understood by Japanese children and maintained the Emotion Detective concept from the original UP-C, which in turn created a fun environment through which they could learn new skills in the treatment program.

Adapting Thinking Trap Characters

In the original UP-C, detectives who tend to fall into each thinking trap appear as thinking trap characters (e.g., the thinking trap of mind reading is referred to as

Psychic Suki), while in the original UP-A, the name of each thinking trap is taught using verbal description. However, in the Japanese version, unique characters, referred to as thinking monsters, were designed to correspond to each thinking trap for both the adapted UP-C and UP-A (Figure 12.1). The purpose of this modification stems from the fact that thinking traps are somewhat difficult for the youth to understand and engage with because they are represented using arcane idioms that are not part of regular everyday lingo in Japan. In addition, within the adapted UP-C, the second skill was renamed the "Culprit Identification" skill to represent the process by which the "culprit" causing difficult emotions is sought out. As a result, the source of the emotional problem had to be externalized as the "culprit" or thinking monster that causes the detective's maladaptive thinking and must be confronted.

When creating each monster, we considered signature phrases that represented their respective thinking traps and based their design on an animal whose name is included in the signature phrase. For example, within the thinking trap for "thinking the worst," *saiaku* is the Japanese word for "worst." Thus, the signature phrase assigned to this thinking trap was "it is the worst!" or *saiakuda!* (note: *da* is an assertive auxiliary verb). As *sai* means "rhinoceros" in English, we created a thinking monster that appears as a villainous rhinoceros named *Saiakku*. Using these associations, remembering the name or signature phrase of each monster is sufficient in aiding recognition of thought patterns that cause difficult emotions, without the need to recall field-specific jargon such as "thinking the worst." As Japanese children love fictional characters such as monsters or *yokai* (mysterious

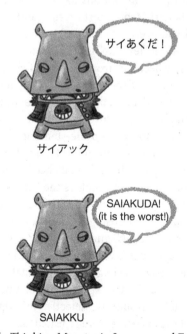

Figure 12.1. Example of a Thinking Monster in Japanese and English

or otherworldly creatures), families were relatively familiar with the external characterization of emotional problems as monsters or *yokai* and readily accepted and understood the concept of thinking monsters. Some children even thought of their own thinking monsters and drew them.

Adapting UP-C/A Worksheets and Forms

In order to properly adapt the UP-C/A worksheets and forms for Japanese clients, we had to consider cross-cultural differences in self-efficacy and their relation to the treatment process. Compared with people in the United States, people in Japan think that they cannot do well when they set high standards for themselves or someone sets high standards for them (Chang et al., 2012). Thus, when the method for completing treatment worksheets or forms is unclear, efficacy and motivation may decrease as clients lose confidence in their ability to engage in the assigned exercises. In tailoring the UP-C/A worksheets to prevent such difficulties, we elucidated the information each worksheet required for accurate completion and added examples for further clarity. A notable example is the "Tracking the Before, During, and After" form, which is referred to as the "Crime Scene Investigation" worksheet in the Japanese adaptation (illustrated in Figure 12.2). To clearly indicate that this form is to be filled out when strong emotions are experienced, the children in the UP-C are prompted to select which emotions they were feeling, while in the UP-A, adolescents simply described their emotions without prompts. For the results section of the form (i.e., what happened after?), in both the UP-C and UP-A, participants selected from *yes* or *no* options for the following questions: "Did that behavior make you feel better?" (short-term result) and "Did that behavior make you 'level up'" (i.e., Did you overcome the problem and become stronger?; long-term result). As the expression "level up" is often used in video games, meaning to advance to the next level or become stronger, it was familiar to Japanese children and enhanced their enjoyment of the worksheet. Only adolescents in the UP-A were asked to provide specific details about the results. In this manner, the difference between short-term and long-term results, which is difficult to understand even for adults, was simplified for better understanding.

For emotion exposures (Sessions 9 through 14 in the UP-C and Module 7 in the UP-A), the original UP-C employs the same "Science Experiment" worksheet used in Session 3, while the original UP-A employs the "Tracking the Before, During, and After" form to track each exposure. We assumed that using one worksheet in multiple manners would be confusing for Japanese youth; thus, we prepared a new "Confrontation" worksheet (Figure 12.3) for Japanese youth to use when tracking exposures. We prepared this worksheet by summarizing the primary steps of exposure from the therapist guide (e.g., rate emotional intensity on the emotion thermometer before, during, and after exposure; predict possible results of the exposure and confirm the actual result; use detective thinking before the exposure; predict possible results if the exposure were repeated) so that the worksheet would guide youth through the same series of steps used in therapy sessions.

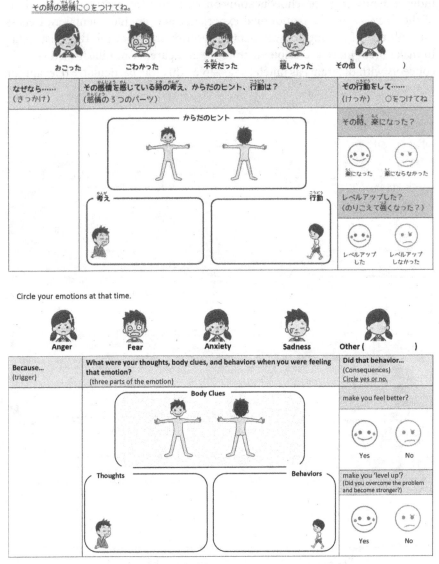

Figure 12.2. Japanese Version of the "Tracking the Before, During, and After" Form in UP-C ("Crime Scene Investigation" Worksheet) in Japanese and English

Adapting the UP-C/A Workbooks

Although the UP-C and UP-A are recommended for use in therapy in Japan as well as in the United States, few organizations or therapists offer CBT in Japan (Takahashi et al., 2018). As a result, many families do not have therapist-guided access to the psychoeducation and skills inherent to the CBT model. With this in mind, we added several figures to both program workbooks to help families lacking access to professional mental health care services learn independently (e.g., psychoeducation on emotions for parents; explanations of the three parts of an emotional experience and nonjudgmental awareness for children). In doing so, we adapted descriptions from the therapist guide to make them more accessible to children and parents and illustrated specific concepts with diagrams as much as possible. This was particularly relevant for adapting the UP-C.

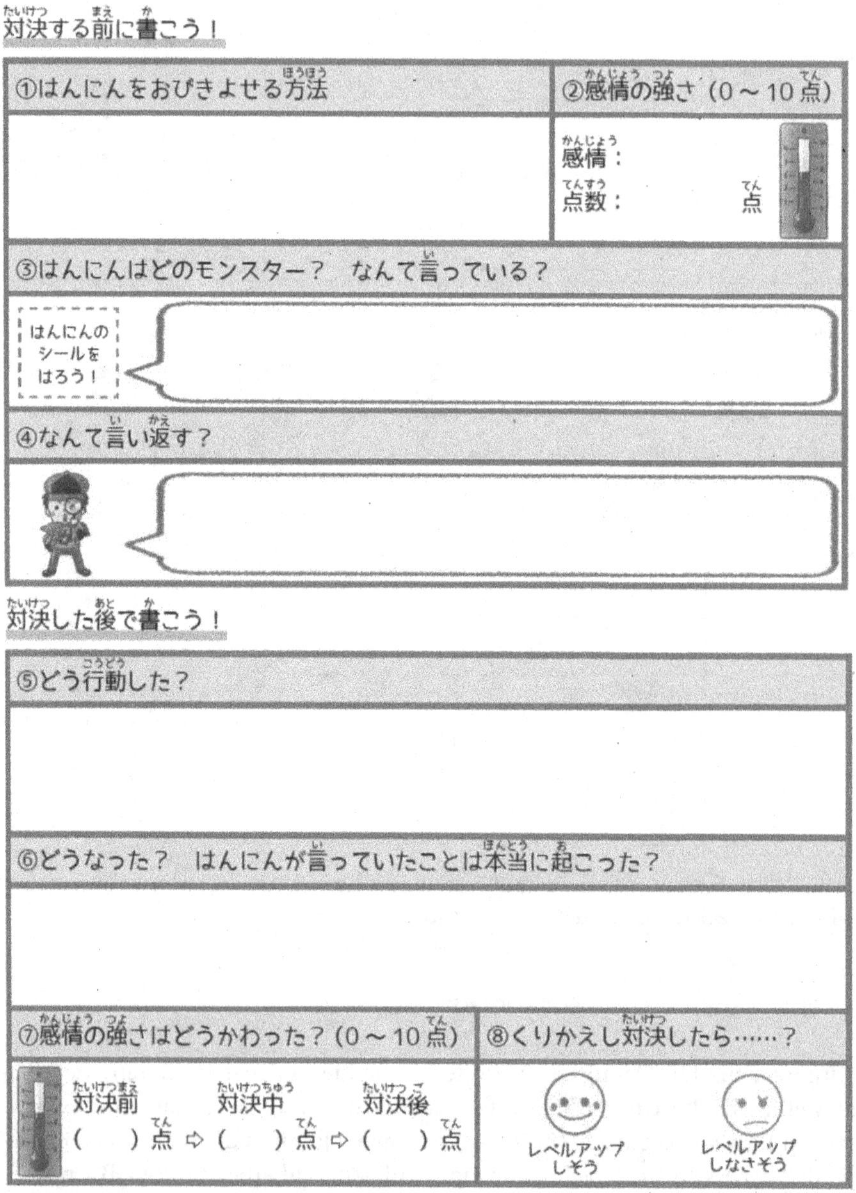

対決する前に書こう！

①はんにんをおびきよせる方法

②感情の強さ（0〜10点）

感情：
点数：　　　　点

③はんにんはどのモンスター？　なんて言っている？

はんにんの
シールを
はろう！

④なんて言い返す？

対決した後で書こう！

⑤どう行動した？

⑥どうなった？　はんにんが言っていたことは本当に起こった？

⑦感情の強さはどうかわった？（0〜10点）

対決前　　　　対決中　　　　対決後
（　　　）点 ⇨ （　　　）点 ⇨ （　　　）点

⑧くりかえし対決したら……？

レベルアップ
しそう

レベルアップ
しなさそう

Figure 12.3. Worksheet for Completing Emotion Exposures in Japanese UP-C in Japanese and English

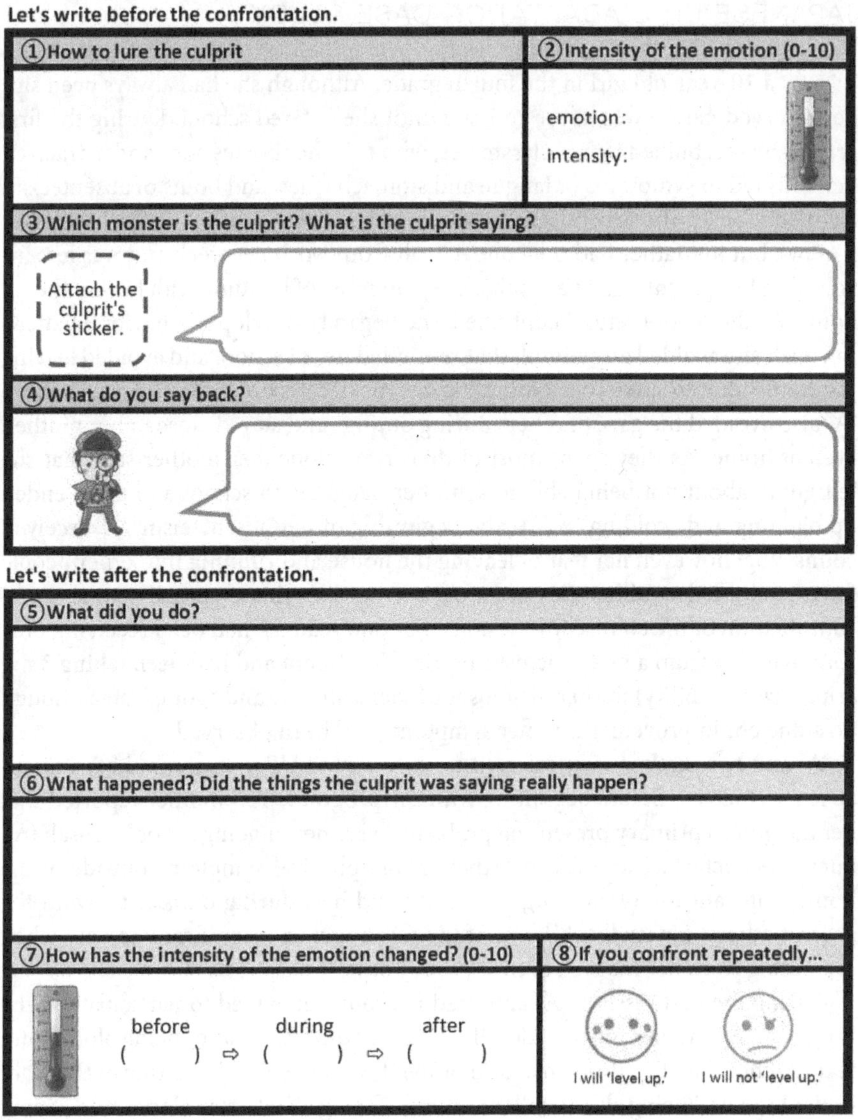

Let's write before the confrontation.

①How to lure the culprit	②Intensity of the emotion (0-10)
	emotion: intensity:

③Which monster is the culprit? What is the culprit saying?
Attach the culprit's sticker.

④What do you say back?

Let's write after the confrontation.

⑤What did you do?

⑥What happened? Did the things the culprit was saying really happen?

⑦How has the intensity of the emotion changed? (0-10)	⑧If you confront repeatedly...
before during after ( ) ⇨ ( ) ⇨ ( )	I will 'level up.' I will not 'level up.'

Figure 12.3. Continued

Furthermore, for Japanese youth lacking access to therapy or mental health support programs, we assumed that learning these treatment protocols would be challenging and sought out ways to make them easier to understand. To that end, in addition to the aforementioned revisions, any words that appeared to be difficult for the youth to comprehend were replaced with simpler, more memorable, and more engaging words. For example, participating in a sensational exposure was called a "body experiment," present-moment awareness was referred to as the "here-and-now mode," and situational emotion exposures were called "confrontations."

JAPANESE UP-C ADAPTATION CASE STUDY

"A" was a 10-year-old girl in the fourth grade. Although she had always been shy, her reserved nature was never an issue until she entered school. During the first grade, she was bullied by her classmates, who took her possessions and ostracized her. This led to symptoms of fatigue and stomachaches, and bouts of absenteeism from school. In the second grade, she mostly stayed home. "A" lived with her parents, but her father had only one day off from work per week and was less involved in her parenting. As a result, she spent most of her time with her mother at home. As the school refusal continued, she began to develop a behavioral pattern in which she avoided any stimuli that reminded her of school and avoided leaving the house due to anxiety surrounding her physical symptoms (stomachaches). "A" also avoided the gaze of others during outings and stayed close to her mother, even at home. As they spent most of their time alone, her mother said that she felt guilty about not being able to send her daughter to school and often ended up blaming and scolding "A." At the beginning of her absenteeism, "A" received counseling; however, her fear of leaving the house and running into other people from school led to difficulties with routine outings. This eventually led to a discontinuation of the counseling sessions. For one year, "A" had been receiving professional help from a pediatric psychiatric department and had been taking 3 mg aripiprazole (Abilify) for her diagnoses of social anxiety and agoraphobia, though no sufficient improvements in her symptoms had been observed.

"A" and her mother were referred to the adapted UP-C program by her pediatric psychiatrist. Before beginning with the program, "A's" mother reported that her daughter's primary presenting problems were her ongoing school refusal; frequent stomachaches and fear of experiencing physical symptoms outside of the home; constant use of clothing (i.e., mask and hat) during outings to avoid the gaze of others, especially children of the same age; and significant anxiety when separating from her mother, even while at home.

During the first session, "A" appeared nervous but agreed to participate in the program. "A" and her mother identified "fear of others," "fear of being alone," and fear of school" as Top Problems for treatment, which led to the setting of three actionable goals: "being able to talk to others," "being able to stay alone," and "being able to go to school."

In the second session, when the "Crime Scene Investigation" worksheet (see Figure 12.2) was introduced, "A" initially appeared hesitant and concerned about making mistakes in completing the form. She was ultimately able to fill out the worksheet by referring to the example provided, and eventually became quite fond of the expression "level up," used in the worksheet to describe the long-term result of overcoming challenging emotional experiences. "A" found this concept particularly engaging, which motivated her to try to "level up" in response to her own difficult emotions. For her Session 2 homework, "A" recorded on her "Crime Scene Investigation" worksheet that she removed her mask and hat while outside and experienced the feeling of "leveling up" as she faced her fear of being seen or recognized by others.

In Session 3, "A" identified various activities, including ones that she used to enjoy such as "going for a walk" and "riding a bicycle," as well as special ones such as "going to the zoo." She was able to practice these activities as behavioral experiments at home. In response to her efforts, her mother reinforced her brave behavior by increasing physical contact and making more time to play together. As "A" responded positively to the reinforcement, her mother noted the effectiveness of the parenting skills taught in the adapted UP-C.

During the body experiment (sensational exposure in the original version) conducted in Session 4, "A" tried spinning for one minute and reported strong physical sensations. With encouragement from her therapist, she was able to carefully observe and identify the feelings in her body. When reflecting on the body experiment, she reported that the uncomfortable physical sensations subsided after some time. She was able to actively engage in the body experiment with her mother as homework. Through this module, "A's" anxiety over her physical sensations gradually reduced. Additionally, "A" recorded on her "Crime Scene Investigation" worksheet that she was able to enter the school building for the first time in two years, albeit for a short period and without other children. Her mother reported that she was able to empathize with "A," who appeared nervous at school.

In Session 5, "A" was very fond of the thinking monsters (see Figure 12.1) from the Culprit Identification skill (the "L" skill in the original version) and accurately identified a personal example for each of the four monsters. Her mother also understood the therapeutic principle well and was able to provide specific scenes wherein each monster appeared for herself and "A."

In Session 6, "A" demonstrated as strong an interest in the Evidence Collection skill (the "detective thinking" aspect of the "U" skill in the original version) as in the Culprit Identification skill. For homework, she was able to complete the "Evidence Collection" worksheet ("U for Children" in the original version) by referring to an example. She reported that *Kimarisu* (the monster of Jumping to Conclusions) told her, "If you go out, you must get a stomachache" but she was able to collect evidence (e.g., "There were times when I went out but didn't get a stomachache") and confirm changes in her thoughts and emotions. Furthermore, she voluntarily told her mother that she wanted to take the train alone and was able to ride on a different car from her mother. Her mother reported that, upon receiving this proposal from "A," she was able to support her by using shaping and positive reinforcement.

"A" reported that through the Strategy Planning skill (the problem-solving aspect of the "U" skill in the original version) she had learned in Session 7, she had been able to talk with her mother about finding a strategy to cope with the problem of having to wait for a few days before seeing a doctor despite having unpleasant symptoms. Her mother also reported that she was able to support "A" in using the Evidence Collection skill and the Strategy Planning skill by using shaping strategies she learned during the previous session. Furthermore, her mother set a goal for "A's" father to play a considerable role in parenting, used the Strategy Planning skill to create a plan for "A's" father to spend more time with

"A," and tried to promote his participation in parenting. Specifically, she decided to have "A" participate in outings on "A's" father's day off and asked him to take on the role of giving "A" reinforcers. Busy fathers in Japan often do not know how to relate to their children, creating a psychological and physical distance between them. Thus, having him take on the role of giving reinforcers increased positive interaction between "A" and her father.

Before using the Confrontation skill (the "E" skill in the original version) in Session 8, "A" told her therapist, "I feel physically better, and I am enjoying going outside." Her mother also reported that "A" was voluntarily taking on challenges more often. "A" performed mindfulness exercises with curiosity, using breathing, snacks, and clay during her sessions and homework, and she learned the importance of focusing on the present moment and not judging her emotions and emotional behaviors. Additionally, her mother included various challenges on the "Confrontation List" (the "Emotional Behavior" form in the original version) on the basis of past challenges, including both those she had not achieved ("go to school while other children are there," "ride a crowded train alone," and "study") and those she had secured a certain degree of mastery on ("go out without the mask and the hat," "go near the school," and "leave mother's side").

Regarding "A's" progress in Sessions 9 through 14, "A" was able to have discussions with her mother, set challenges, and achieve the following: "study and go to school to report to the teacher," "read a book report out loud in front of the teacher," "order food by herself at a fast-food restaurant and eat the food as a reward," and "go to a movie theater or tourist spots at a distant location." On the "Confrontation" worksheet (see Figure 12.3), she applied her favorite skills: Culprit Identification and Evidence Collection. When going to school, she said *Omitoushi* (the monster of Mind Reading) was telling her "other children would think of her as being strange." When going to a fast-food restaurant, she said *Kimarisu* told her "you will run into some kids you know who will try to talk to you." When going far, *Kimarisu* told her "you will get sick." She was able to challenge each thought (e.g., "No one is going to think that," "If someone talks to me, I just have to say I came here for lunch," and "I will be fine, as my condition is improving"). During the sessions, with the therapist's encouragement, she was able to achieve challenges such as "reading a book report in front of a group of guardians," "shopping at a convenience store without the mask and the hat," and "not wearing the mask and the hat during sessions." Through these challenges, "A" learned that negative predictions are not very likely to come true, that she would become comfortable after a while even if she was nervous at the beginning, and that she is able to manage her anxiety. Additionally, her mother realized that she was attempting to make the challenges easier ahead of time and frequently asking "Are you OK?" while supporting "A" in confrontations, and she was able to gradually correct these overprotective behavioral patterns. Furthermore, her mother reported that by inviting "A's" father on outings, she was pleased to see more opportunities for her father to participate in parenting.

During the final session, "A" said, "It was great to identify thinking monsters, think about the different possibilities, and confront them through this program.

Because of this program, I am now able to remove the mask and the hat, and even go to school. I want to keep taking on many challenging things in the future." Her new goal was "to go to school more often." Her mother reported that "A" was spontaneously using the Culprit Identification, Evidence Collection, Strategy Planning, and Confrontation skills and said that she actively used opposite parenting behaviors to support A's confrontations. The self-reported Spence Children's Anxiety Scale (Spence, 1998) total score for "A" was 71 before the intervention, 38 during the intervention, and 23 after the intervention. At the three-month follow-up, her score improved to 19. Her mother's parent-report score on the same evaluation was 80 before the intervention, 44 during the intervention, and 35 after the intervention; it was 29 at the three-month follow-up.

CONCLUSION

We introduced specific steps for the cultural adaptation of the UP-C and the UP-A in Japan. When introducing the UP-C/A to a Japanese context, modifications were made to increase the acceptability and boost understanding of the treatment, though no significant modifications were made to the content of the intervention protocol. During the preliminary trial in Japan, the adapted UP-C was found to have a low dropout rate and to have reduced the overall severity of psychopathology and functional impairment in clients, thus presenting promising results for the dissemination and implementation of the treatment to new cultural settings. A clinical trial using the adapted UP-A is currently in preparation. In the future, as the UP-C/A is introduced to additional cultures and treatment settings, its effectiveness will be further assessed and the cultural adaptations necessary to serve new cultural groups will become increasingly clear.

Tip Sheet for Using UP-C and UP-A in Youth in the Context of Other Cultures

✓ Why use culturally adapted UP-C and UP-A in the context of other cultures?
  - Previous studies showed that culturally and linguistically adapted psychotherapy is more effective than unadapted psychotherapy.
  - It is important for therapists to maintain a balance between scientifically rigorous interventions and culturally competent practice.
  - The UP-C and UP-A are transdiagnostic treatments that target emotion dysregulation rather than specific disorders. Therefore, these treatments may be more readily amenable to adaptation for other cultures, especially those with higher levels of stigma surrounding psychological disorders and psychiatric diagnoses.

✓ How do I use UP-C and UP-A in the context of other cultures?
  - When introducing the UP-C and UP-A into a new cultural context, it is important to consider that direct translation may not be sufficient and systematic modification may be needed in some countries and regions.
  - For example, in Japan, program and skill names were changed, and "thinking monsters" were created in place of the original thinking trap characters. Additionally, worksheets and other materials were adapted for use with Japanese youth to account for the cultural context.

✓ What challenges might come up when using UP-C and UP-A in the context of other cultures?
  - CBT may not be widely available in non-Western countries, including Japan; thus, many families may not have access to therapists or organizations that are familiar with the psychoeducation and skills inherent to the CBT model. It may be helpful to add some materials to provide detailed descriptions to the UP-C and UP-A workbooks to help these families learn independently.

✓ When is the UP-C or UP-A not appropriate in the context of other cultures?
  - In cultures where the basic principles of the intervention could be accepted, it is likely that UP-C or UP-A would be appropriate. However, further ingenuity may be required when introducing them to cultures with low literacy rates as they often use worksheets that require reading and writing.

REFERENCES

American Psychological Association Presidential Task Force on Evidence-Based Practice in Psychology. (2006). Evidence-based practice in psychology. *American Psychologist, 61*, 271–285.

Ando, S., Yamaguchi, S., Aoki, Y., & Thornicroft, G. (2013). Review of mental-health-related stigma in Japan. *Psychiatry and Clinical Neurosciences, 67*(7), 471–482.

Benish, S. G., Quintana, S., & Wampold, B. E. (2011). Culturally adapted psychotherapy and the legitimacy of myth: A direct-comparison meta-analysis. *Journal of Counseling Psychology, 58*(3), 279–289.

Bernal, G., Jiménez-Chafey, M. I., & Domenech Rodríguez, M. D. (2009). Cultural adaptation of treatments: A resource for considering culture in evidence-based practice. *Professional Psychology: Research and Practice, 40*, 361–368.

Chang, E. C., Chang, R., & Sanna, L. J. (2012). A test of the usefulness of perfectionism theory across cultures: Does perfectionism in the US and Japan predict depressive symptoms across time? *Cognitive Therapy and Research, 36*(1), 1–14.

Griner, D., & Smith, T.B. (2006). Culturally adapted mental health intervention: A meta-analytic review. *Psychotherapy, 43*(4), 531–548.

Hays, P. A. (2009). Integrating evidence-based practice, cognitive–behavior therapy, and multicultural therapy: Ten steps for culturally competent practice. *Professional Psychology: Research and Practice, 40*(4), 354–360.

Hinton, D. E., & Patel, A. (2017). Cultural adaptations of cognitive behavioral therapy. *Psychiatric Clinics of North America, 40*(4), 701–714.

Masuda, A., Hayes, S., Twohig, M., Lillis, J., Fletcher, L., & Gloster, A. (2009). Comparing Japanese international college students' and U.S. college students' mental-health-related stigmatizing attitudes. *Journal of Multicultural Counseling and Development, 37*(3), 178–189.

Spence, S. H. (1998). A measure of anxiety symptoms among children. *Behaviour Research and Therapy, 36*(5), 545–566.

Takahashi, F., Takegawa, S., Okumura, Y., & Suzuki, S. (2018). Actual condition survey on the implementation of cognitive behavioral therapy at psychiatric clinics in Japan [in Japanese]. http://ftakalab.jp/wordpress/wp-content/uploads/2011/08/japancbtclinic_report.pdf

Yoshioka, K., Reavley, N. J., MacKinnon, A. J., & Jorm, A. F. (2014). Stigmatising attitudes towards people with mental disorders: Results from a survey of Japanese high school students. *Psychiatry Research, 215*(1), 229–236.

Tables, figures and boxes are indicated by *t*, *f* and *b* following the page number